PRAISE FOR TO BE ALIVE

"This is a practical and hopeful guide for women of all ages who have been diagnosed with cancer, providing accurate information, perceptive support, and useful advice. *To Be Alive* offers crucial help to women cancer survivors and lets them know they are not alone."
—Diane Blum, M.S.W., executive director of Cancer Care, Inc.

"*To Be Alive* gives insight and advice that can only come from one who has journeyed through the diagnosis of cancer and the battle to overcome it. Dr. Carolyn Runowicz made that journey. She is also a cancer specialist, so she is uniquely qualified to offer helpful and much-needed information to women cancer survivors."
—Penny Wise Budoff, M.D., author of *No More Hot Flashes and Other Good News*

"Written with a rare blend of professional knowledge and personal experience, *To Be Alive* will help women unravel the mysteries of life after cancer. It offers tools that promote awareness and responsibility so that women can optimize their chances for full recovery."
— Susan Leigh, R.N., cancer survivorship consultant and president of the National Coalition for Cancer Survivorship

To Be Alive

A WOMAN'S GUIDE TO A FULL LIFE AFTER CANCER

· · · · ·

Carolyn D. Runowicz, M.D.
and Donna Haupt

HENRY HOLT AND COMPANY · NEW YORK

Henry Holt and Company, Inc.
Publishers since 1866
115 West 18th Street
New York, New York 10011

Henry Holt® is a registered
trademark of Henry Holt and Company, Inc.

Copyright © 1995 by Carolyn D. Runowicz, M.D.
All rights reserved.
Published in Canada by Fitzhenry & Whiteside Ltd.,
195 Allstate Parkway, Markham, Ontario L3R 4T8.

Library of Congress Cataloging-in-Publication Data
Runowicz, Carolyn D.
To be alive: a woman's guide to a full life after cancer /
Carolyn D. Runowicz and Donna Haupt.—1st ed.
p. cm.
Includes index.
1. Cancer—Popular works. 2. Women—Diseases. 3. Generative
organs, Female—Cancer. 4. Breast—Cancer. 5. Cancer—
Psychological aspects. I. Haupt, Donna. II. Title.
RC281.W65R86 1995 94-49435
616.99406—dc20 CIP

ISBN 0-8050-2958-3
ISBN 0-8050-2959-1 (An Owl Book: pbk.)

Henry Holt books are available for special promotions
and premiums. For details contact: Director, Special Markets.

First published in hardcover in 1995 by
Henry Holt and Company, Inc.

First Owl Book Edition—1996

Designed by Victoria Hartman

Printed in the United States of America
All first editions are printed on acid-free paper.∞

1 3 5 7 9 10 8 6 4 2
1 3 5 7 9 10 8 6 4 2 (pbk.)

*To my husband,
for all his unending
love and support
during my darkest days*

· CONTENTS ·

Acknowledgments xi
Preface xiii

One · Loss of Innocence: My Story as a Survivor 1
Two · Putting Treatment Behind You 10
Three · The Need for Follow-up Care 27
Four · Taking Care of Your Health:
Diet, Nutrition, and Lifestyle 37
Five · Coping with Physical Scars 66
Six · Sex After Cancer 89
Seven · The Road to Motherhood 113
Eight · Cancer's Effect on the Family 132
Nine · Facing Menopause 144
Ten · Stress, Loneliness, and Depression 163
Eleven · Fear of Recurrence and Second Cancers 175
Twelve · Job and Insurance Discrimination 201

Afterword · Where Do We Go from Here? 227
Support Groups and Resources 229
Index 241

· ACKNOWLEDGMENTS ·

Dr. Carolyn Runowicz would like to thank her medical oncologist, Dr. Larry Norton, and her surgeon, Dr. Michail Shafir, for their constant support and wonderful care. She is grateful to her colleagues Dr. Gary Goldberg and Dr. Harriet Smith for maintaining patient care and the practice. She also thanks Bea Mussolini for her secretarial assistance and support.

Donna Haupt would like to thank her editors and colleagues at *Life* magazine for showing her what good and responsible journalism should be. She is grateful to the many survivors and medical experts who spoke with her so openly and contributed their experience and advice. She also thanks her mother for instilling in her a love of medicine and showing her that cancer, though sometimes deadly, is a disease that can be fought with dignity and enormous strength. Finally, she thanks her husband, Amir, and son, Matthew, for enough things to fill a hundred books, but most of all for reminding her, one day at a time, that they knew she could do it.

· PREFACE ·

Cancer-free. Survivor. Impossible notions only a few decades ago. Now these words have an exquisite sweetness, a euphoria grounded in the fierce determination of survivors and their families to continue with the business of living. By the year 2000 the American Cancer Society estimates ten million Americans will be cancer survivors. Of the seven million today, more than half are women who have triumphed over their disease. No matter where their cancer first struck, or what their ultimate prognosis, their survival began the day their treatment ended. Now they face a still greater challenge of reaffirming within themselves the power of life—of beginning again.

When a woman first learns she has cancer, she and her loved ones turn to the oncologist for information about her illness, leaning on the combined strength of her medical support team for direction and encouragement in the demanding fight simply to stay alive. Many books now document this battle, some the heartrending stories of women we all know: Gilda Radner, Betty Rollin, Ann Jillian. Their courage and dignity have helped those diagnosed with cancer to bear the burden of treatment, to persevere.

But the woman who *survives* cancer faces rocky, uncharted territory. Often she must contend with the disabling consequences of therapy and face ongoing concerns about living with a frightening, chronic disease. Slowly she begins to realize that her body may not look, feel, or function exactly the way it did prior to her illness. And she may find herself reevaluating her relationships, her career, her goals, even her sense of purpose. On top of this comes the ever-present threat of recurrence, a fear that stalks, to varying degrees, every cancer survivor.

Several years ago I started out to write a book for survivors that would share my professional knowledge and experience as an oncologist who has treated women for cancer over the past fifteen years. I wanted to offer women a source book filled with medical information and tangible advice on how to enter the "well world" again. I knew—from an intellectual standpoint, that is—the range of anxiety and frustration cancer could heap on a patient and her family.

But in July 1992, when I discovered a lump in my own left breast, the book project went on hold. I had breast cancer. And it would take a year of grueling therapy before I too could face forward, a survivor—feeling in my heart what it means to begin life again. As my own experience taught me, no single resource specifically addressed the postrecovery fears, emotions, and physical concerns of women who have survived cancer. No guide existed to help women navigate the obstacles of lost friendships, diminished investment options, and job discrimination that might ensue after having had cancer.

As survivors, women deserved a book that showed them how to maintain their health, how to prevent recurrence, and how to regain physical, emotional, and economic autonomy over their lives. So with the unique perspective of a survivor *and* an oncologist, I decided to write *To Be Alive*, the first book of its kind to help women like myself heal their lives.

Although written specifically for survivors, *To Be Alive* extends beyond that audience. I wanted my own story of survival and those of my patients to act as catalysts for honest conversations about the cancer experience, not only among survivors, but also between wives and husbands, mothers and daughters, friends and co-workers, women and their caregivers.

Perhaps most important, I wanted women to know they were not alone, that others shared their experience, their thoughts and feelings. Although each survivor will have to struggle in her own way to regain the parts of the woman she was, and work to accept her altered version as victor over the disease, she shouldn't have to suffer in isolation.

There can be joy in beginning again, an excitement that comes from making every minute count. If this book makes that happen for just a few survivors who read it, I know I've done my job.

To Be Alive

One

LOSS OF INNOCENCE: MY STORY AS A SURVIVOR

From the moment I discovered the lump, my life was never the same. It happened the last weekend of June 1992. My husband and I had arrived late the night before at our summer house on Shelter Island, stealing away for three days together to walk on the beach, barbecue for friends, and clear our minds. I was an oncologist and Sheldon an obstetrician, each of us with a demanding New York City practice, so we relished the chance, no matter how brief, to pause our hectic lives and hear nothing but the sounds of the bay beyond our bedroom deck.

Sheldon volunteered to make coffee that morning, letting me linger a bit longer in the shower. As the water cascaded off my back, I spread a thin lather of soap across my chest, slowly circling the muscles above my heart. It was a quick exam I practiced each month after my period, a routine I'd advised all my patients to do. But when my fingers paused on a small, pea-size ball beneath the skin of my left breast, I froze. No, I thought. It's just a cyst. It'll be gone by tomorrow.

But the next morning, when I examined myself, the lump was still there. It lay in the left upper, outer quadrant, the most common place for a breast cancer to occur. Like most tumors, it was hard and didn't separate from the tissue surrounding it. And though I was young, only forty-one, the fact was I'd never had children and had taken birth control pills for many years, both risk factors for the disease.

Still, I had always considered myself exempt. I'd devoted my life

1

to healing others, rising through the ranks of a male-dominated profession to become director of gynecologic oncology at Albert Einstein College of Medicine and Montefiore Medical Center, one of the country's leading medical institutions. Over the past fifteen years I'd become an authority on the disease, writing countless articles for medical journals and national magazines about its prevention and treatment in women. I knew where cancer started and how it could end. But I never thought it would strike out at me.

The next day my mammogram came back negative. Though part of me was relieved, I knew that in young women like myself, the density of the breast tissue could sometimes mask evidence of disease. To be certain, I needed a biopsy.

The Race to Be Cured

The pathologist's office was in midtown Manhattan, its waiting room crowded with women awaiting diagnosis. I had packed my briefcase with paperwork, figuring I might have to wait. But each time they called a new patient, I looked up, wondering whether my name would be next. It felt odd to be on this side of the fence, knowing that within the hour cells would be drawn from the nodule in my breast and examined under the microscope, confirming on the spot whether I had cancer or not.

When my turn finally came, I was led to a tiny, windowless examining room and told to undress. Lying back on a padded table, I draped a sheet across my chest and tried to stay calm. The procedure was painful but quick, the pathologist reassuring me throughout that I had nothing to worry about.

"I'll develop it for you right away so you'll know," she said, and left for a moment. But as I finished getting dressed, she poked her head in, asking me to come back to her office.

At once my antennae went up. Why hadn't she told me then, instead of asking me to her office? Taking a seat, I searched her eyes for a clue.

"It looks suspicious," she said, meeting my gaze.

"So I'll get another opinion."

"No, I'm really sorry," she said, shaking her head slowly. "It's definitely cancer."

At that point the room went blank. I felt this strangling, choking feeling, that I had to get air, to get to the street. And as I ran through the waiting room, the receptionist called after me, "Wait. You didn't pay your bill."

I think I found a cab to take me home. I can't remember. There were so many things now to worry about. The cancer was still small enough to warrant lumpectomy with radiation, but I needed to act fast. I telephoned the surgeon who trained me, someone whose expertise I trusted. And by luck he was in that afternoon.

"You're not going to believe this," I said, trying to control my panic, "but I just had a needle aspiration done on my left breast and it's positive. You've got to operate on me tomorrow."

He agreed.

That evening Sheldon sat beside me in our kitchen as I called all the patients I had booked for surgery the next day and over the following few weeks. When I told them one of my associates would be taking over because I too needed cancer surgery, some began to cry, afraid that I would die and leave them in the lurch. I remember one husband actually said, "Oh, I wish you'd discovered that lump next week." He apologized later, saying he hadn't meant it. But of course he had. He wanted his wife cared for first, not me.

My surgery the next day went smoothly. As I dozed in and out of twilight sleep in the recovery room, my mind began to plan my visits to radiation therapy. Somehow I was under the illusion that I would come out of surgery and be back on my feet the following week. I hadn't thought about the possibility of dying. I simply told myself,

Okay, the tumor was less than a centimeter and I have no palpable nodes. Once this thing is removed, I'm out of here. Back to my life, just the way it always has been.

But when I tried to get out of my hospital bed the next morning, a searing pain shot through my chest. A plastic drain had been sutured under my armpit, making it impossible to move my left arm, even in the slightest.

"What about helping me get dressed so I can get out of here?" I said to the private duty nurse by my bedside.

"But it's five in the morning, and your doctor hasn't come in."

"Either you help me or I'll do it myself," I countered, grimacing with pain. "I know I'll be better off in my own bed."

But when I got home I was miserable. It was a cold and wet July Fourth weekend. Every time I tried to move, I screamed from the pain. For three solid days the rain poured down, as if the sky had opened up and was sobbing. And though Sheldon would come into the bedroom, offering tea or to brush my hair, I knew he felt helpless. At one point, in a feeble attempt to stay in control, I told him how sorry I was that the radiation treatments were going to spoil our summer. But it never entered my mind how terrified he must have been of losing me.

The Bad News

Days later I began to regroup. The shock of finding cancer, followed by surgery and its painful aftermath, had side-railed my life. I knew radiation treatments would confine my schedule a bit, but I was determined to see patients and keep my busy schedule. Cancer had become an inconvenience, a minor glitch in my plans, but it was not going to rule my life.

Then my surgeon called.

"Carolyn, I'll get right to the point," he said. "The pathology report's come back, and it shows lymphovascular invasion and positive lymph nodes."

Cancer had spread to my lymph nodes, inching its way into my bloodstream and beyond. Like a bomb going off in my brain, the fear took hold. The back pain, the shoulder ache. It all made sense now.

I'm dead, I thought. It's in my spine and I'll never survive. I'm descending into a deep, bottomless black hole.

Fortunately my bone scan came back negative, showing no signs of metastasis. I had finally found the bottom of the hole—no more bad news. But still I needed chemotherapy, a series of twelve treatments once every three weeks, to assure no wayward cancer cells took hold. All along I'd thought I was in control. Now I knew it was cancer that held the reins.

The Price of Survival

Overnight, survival became my one and only goal. I stopped taking on new patients, and I decreased my operating schedule to once a week at most. Although I still kept office hours, I tried to leave by three in the afternoon. I canceled most of my commitments on national committees and found replacement speakers for the lectures I'd promised to give. I simply wasn't sure I could deliver. Every time I had a chemotherapy treatment, it not only killed the cancer cells, it depressed my immune system, interfering with my body's natural ability to fight off infection. If my white blood cell count dropped too low, any sneeze or sniffle near me could spell disaster. I couldn't take airplanes or be in crowded rooms. Quite simply, the bottom had fallen out of my career.

Although I felt sad for myself, I never fell apart. I guess that's because I believed in what I did as an oncologist. I believed that chemotherapy could work and that you didn't have to die from breast cancer. Having cancer in my lymph nodes clearly skewed the odds, but I never let that defeat me. It wasn't optimism, it was survival—a belief that others might die, but not me.

By August my hair started to fall out. I was sitting on the deck at Shelter Island, running a brush through my scalp, when huge clumps began to blow off into the wind. "Prepare yourself," I said out loud. "You're going to look in the mirror and be bald." But it's amazing how much hair you have on your head. It ended up taking a good two weeks before I'd lost it all.

The nausea was something else. Once a month, after three hours on an intravenous drip, I would barely make it home before the spasms ripped through my insides, sending me retching to the bathroom for hours. I'd spend the rest of the weekend sleeping, waking sometime in midafternoon to the distant sound of traffic below in the street. Once when I awakened, the bedroom was hot and stuffy, and a thin layer of sweat had accumulated on my skin. As I padded past the front door, Sheldon's key entered the lock. I must have looked terrible, standing there in my terry-cloth bathrobe, my face gaunt, my eyes sunken, just a few strands of hair left. But he hugged me as if nothing had changed and guided me gently to the living room couch.

"You're halfway through," he said, handing me a neatly wrapped box from Tiffany's. That was Sheldon's way. Throughout this ordeal he had showered me with gifts, never complaining, never faltering in his resolve to care for me, to make me feel special, to be there for support.

Inside the box were two gold disks, rimmed with silver, and a necklace to match. I remember holding them up to my ears and closing my eyes. Then I jerked up. The sun had gone down, and there was a red glow to the room. The table was set, and food smells wafted from the kitchen. I had fallen back asleep.

Somehow I managed to get through the chemotherapy and still see my patients. Some noticed my wig and would say, "Your hair really looks different." When I told them why, there would be a stunned silence. Many of them thought that if I died, they would, too. And they cried and were afraid. Some sent me reams of literature on shark cartilage and herbal tea remedies. Others fixed me frozen dinners to take home at night.

Getting through office hours took every ounce of energy I had left. I'd examine a patient and discuss her progress, then retreat to my office, where my nurses fed me orange juice to stave off the weakness and the nausea. One day, as I struggled to hoist myself out of my chair, the chairman of the department came in.

"It's ridiculous to work when you feel so miserable," he said, sounding more than a little concerned.

"I'll be fine," I said, too exhausted to argue.

"Now listen, no one expects you to be here," he persisted. "What are you trying to prove?"

In a way he was right, but in order to heal myself I needed to feel some semblance of normalcy in my life.

Eight months into my ordeal, chemotherapy stopped and my radiation treatments began. I was fitted for a body mold to immobilize me during therapy, and my chest was tattooed with little black dots so that the nozzle of the radiation machine lined up exactly with my tumor. The walls of the room were two feet thick and lined with lead. And though the technicians were very nice, explaining every adjustment they made, I was terrified. From the moment they turned to close the vaultlike door behind them, it was all I could do not to run behind them, screaming.

All these crazy thoughts went through my head: What if the beam starts to shake and hits my eyes? What if I breathe too deeply and the radiation hits the wrong spot? Even though I was a doctor and knew the chances were slim, I still felt that fear every time I went in.

Day of Reckoning

As suddenly as cancer started, my treatments ended. It was Memorial Day 1993, and though I would continue to see my doctors every three months, it felt as though an umbilical cord had been cut. When you're under treatment, you're too busy to think. Almost every week there's a blood count to get or some interaction with your medical team. Then one day it's over and you're on your own.

I now was in "clinical remission," a stage where the longer I went without a recurrence, the greater my chances were of staying cured. On the Saturday of July Fourth weekend, Sheldon and I went out to Shelter Island to celebrate the first anniversary of my diagnosis and the conclusion of my treatments. His children had come, and at dinner that evening my stepdaughter toasted me, saying, "You taught us how to be an inspiration, how to get over this ordeal with dignity and with strength."

But the truth was, I wasn't really over it. I had just begun to face up to what I'd been through. While they boasted about how good I looked and how great it must feel to put cancer behind me, the fact was I looked lousy and felt even worse. When I looked in the mirror, I saw an old woman staring back at me, a strand of hair here and there, with no eyebrows, no eyelashes, a prisoner of war. My clothes hung on a bony frame. And at forty-two I'd begun to suffer the hot flashes and vaginal dryness that come from premature menopause.

Over dinner that evening I snapped at Sheldon for overcooking the swordfish. I complained that the wine was too warm. No one seemed in tune with what I was feeling, and that made me feel empty, isolated. Not until months later, when one of my patients, a lawyer, told me how she'd taken a nosedive on her anniversary and ended up needing antidepressant medication, did I begin to understand the mystery of my own emotions.

As happens with so many cancer survivors, my first anniversary became a day of reckoning. I had the rest of my life in front of me, but all my options had changed. If I wanted to further my medical career and teach at another university, I had to consider my insurance options as well as my career. If I wanted to buy more life insurance, I couldn't. Cancer gave me a preexisting medical condition that no insurance carrier was prepared to take on.

All the personal landmarks I might have missed—listening to the squeals of my four-year-old nephew, watching Sheldon's granddaughter blow out her birthday candles—came flooding before my eyes. I had lost my innocence, and in the fullest sense I realized how very close I'd come to my own mortality.

About a month later my hair began to come in. Although I looked like Sinéad O'Connor, the very fact that there was fuzz on my head signaled the beginning of my rebirth. Slowly the fatigue lifted, and I knew I needed to start tackling the many issues that faced me as a cancer survivor.

There had been no formal exit from sick to well, no instruction sheet on what to do next with my life. Cancer was my "trial by fire." In surviving it, I had learned many precious lessons. Perhaps one of the most important: Staying alive is just the initial challenge; living with the consequences of the disease and therapy becomes a lifelong responsibility.

Two

PUTTING TREATMENT BEHIND YOU

*F*inishing treatment is a landmark event, a time of relief and celebration for every cancer patient and her family. Yet all too often women find themselves unprepared for the avalanche of emotions that can hit once therapy has ended. For many there is a sense of ambivalence and confusion: on the one hand, they feel joy that their cancer has been stopped, yet they are also fearful of distancing themselves from the health care team that has helped them reach this point of survival.

For twelve long months Shelly endured her chemotherapy as though it were a prison sentence, marking off each course on her calendar with the words "If I can just get through the next round, I'll be okay." Although the cancer in her ovary had been discovered early, doctors still advised chemotherapy to ward off any spread of the disease. Dutifully she'd submitted, somehow managing to run her mail-order food business between the grueling bouts of nausea, the diarrhea, and the lowering blood counts that ensued after every course of therapy. "To get myself through it, I'd dream what it would be like to leave the hospital for the very last time," remembers the forty-two-year-old mother of three. "I looked forward to how happy I'd be and how good the world would look."

But when that time actually came, Shelly found herself more frightened than elated. "I remember my doctor coming in and saying, 'Get dressed, Shelly, you're going home.' But instead of feeling great,

I felt this terrible sense of isolation. It was as if I'd been thrown into a massive ocean without a life preserver and told to swim to shore."

No matter how loathsome their experience with treatment, most women find the demands of therapy in some way reassuring. At least I'm doing something to fight my cancer, they tell themselves, struggling for eight, twelve, sometimes eighteen months of their lives to withstand its rigors. Many have had frequent, if not daily, contact with a team of medical professionals, relying on their expertise for support and guidance in an allied fight against a deadly disease. So when treatment finally ends, and their line of defense is severed, it's only natural for survivors to feel a mass of conflicting emotions.

At this critical juncture, the reality of reentering the "well world" can seem overwhelming. I know as a cancer patient myself, I was so busy being sick, and trying to get well, that I never considered what the rest of my life would be like once—and if—I reached remission. I was consumed with getting through the next hurdle, the next round of chemotherapy, the next stage of radiation. First there were twelve treatments, then eleven, then ten . . . until suddenly my doctor congratulated me on a battle well fought and left me with the words "See you in three months."

Like many survivors, I felt the need for closure, for some informal debriefing session where I could sit down with my team of doctors and go over what I'd been through and what to expect. But this rarely, if ever, occurs.

"Those first few weeks after treatment I felt shell-shocked," says Miriam, an economics professor in upstate New York who developed cancer at age forty-five. "All around me people were congratulating me, saying how great it must be to have completed treatment. But instead of being happy, all I felt was numb. The social worker at the hospital told me this was a common reaction, but I still had a hard time understanding why."

Letting go of treatment and learning to rebuild your life is never an easy journey. While some women seem to make the trip from patient to survivor without too much trouble, others find every step an uphill battle. The road to good health and emotional well-being will differ from woman to woman. But knowing where the potholes and pratfalls are along the way can help you find your path home safely.

Understanding Your Emotions

Gail was one of those take-charge women who'd always prided herself on being in control of her life. She'd set goals for herself and achieved each one, rising through the ranks of her law firm to achieve partner status at the unheard-of age of thirty-six. When she developed ovarian cancer three weeks shy of her forty-ninth birthday, she struggled to maintain control, scheduling her chemotherapy treatments between appearances in court. Every minute of every day was taken up either fighting the cancer or trying to catch up at work, until one morning I visited her hospital room to tell her she was through. Her treatments had been successful, and Gail was at last cancer-free.

Because the chemotherapy had left her exhausted and severely immunodepressed, I advised her to stay at home for several weeks. She'd arrange to have her work sent to her apartment by courier until her white blood cell counts returned to normal.

"There's no keeping this gal down," she told me cheerfully when I came to bid her good-bye.

"Call me in a week to let me know how you're doing," I told her.

And I watched as she sprinted to the elevator, eager and determined to get on with her life.

But when three weeks went by and I still hadn't heard from her, I called her home. The small, almost childlike voice that spoke into the phone was one I hardly recognized.

"I just couldn't handle the memories," she explained tearfully. On the anniversary of her diagnosis, she'd found herself alone and isolated in an empty loft apartment, staring at herself in the mirror. "Every time I try to charge myself up about being alive, I realize how changed my life has become. Everything looks different to me, and all I can do is cry."

Like many cancer survivors, Gail needed time to mourn her life before cancer, to grieve over the fact that after cancer things are never quite the same. Having cancer changes you as an individual in a multitude of ways—some so intangible that it's impossible to articulate them, others visible and apparent by the scars that are left behind.

Each woman must work through her feelings of sadness and loneliness, isolation and fear, in her own private way. One day may bring feelings of confidence, the next day despair. As another patient of mine, Sylvia, came to learn, the mind can sometimes take much longer to recover from cancer than the body.

"When I stopped being a patient and turned into a survivor, I was one giant mass of fears. How would I pay for my treatments? Would I lose my job benefits? Would I get adequate follow-up care? My body had changed, and I worried whether I'd ever get my energy back, if the residual disabilities I now had would prevent me from doing certain things. I worried about being too dependent on my family, whether the stress of my illness would make my family sick, how much I should tell them about what I was thinking, whether the cancer I'd had put them at risk as well. All this contributed to my feeling isolated, even shunned by some friends.

"By the time my hair started to grow back in the second month after the treatment, my moods started to lift a bit. But it really took a full year before my mind caught up with my body and I felt like a well person again."

Some degree of depression following treatment is normal for all cancer survivors. Studies have shown that while major mental illness is uncommon, cancer survivors do have an increased incidence of emotional problems in coping with the trauma of their disease, which tends to disrupt the task of easing back to a normal daily existence.

When I brought this up at a recent meeting of a survivors' support group, one of my patients made an interesting comparison: facing down cancer is in many ways like living through a natural disaster. She had located a research paper by UCLA psychologist Linda Nelson, Ph.D., who studied people involved in more than twenty natural disasters over the past sixty years. Dr. Nelson's conclusion:

> Residents in the stricken communities generally keep their heads, care for one another, share common resources, and actually reach an emotional high as they pull together and tackle the common challenges of survival and rebuilding. Many of them feel saddened at some level when the crisis is over; they realize that they have never experienced that emotion before and perhaps never will [again].

No woman can come through an experience as traumatic as cancer without changing. On the positive side, many survivors have told me that once they have grieved their life before cancer, they have actually come to see a beneficial side to their illness. Rita, a forty-nine-year-old accountant and mother of three grown children, described it this way:

"Hard as it is to say, getting cancer may have been the best thing to happen to me. I spent most of my adult life consumed by my job. I had a husband, children, and a great group of friends, but rather than be a wife or mother or friend back to them, I was a drone. I'd work fourteen-hour days and bring home paperwork on weekends. When cancer came along, I started to look at my loved ones differently. Now, when we're together I'm filled with this indescribable joy. And their concern for my well-being makes me happier than I've ever felt. If I hadn't gotten cancer, I'm not sure I would ever have learned to feel and express love in the same way."

The experience of cancer often leads many survivors to critically review their values and life's priorities. In confronting their own mortality through sickness and the hard-fought struggle for health, many women find they are better able to accept both themselves and the smaller glitches in life. Fitzhugh Mullan, M.D. a pediatrician and chairman of the National Coalition for Cancer Survivorship, calls this reorientation "life rekindled."

Yet this process of learning to accept life is sometimes side-railed by small, seemingly harmless events.

Jerilyn, a petite, blond-haired store manager from central New Jersey, first experienced symptoms of her cervical cancer when she went to visit her in-laws at their oceanfront beach house. Now three years cancer-free, she cannot return to the vacation home without feeling depressed and anxious.

"I walk in the door and the smell of the place, its overall feel, brings back memories of my cancer," Jerilyn explained. "And every time I go to the shore, I can't help thinking I'm going to die, or get sick again."

Sometimes it's hard to point a finger at why you're feeling angry or scared. Lena, an ovarian cancer patient I treated with a hysterectomy and chemotherapy, visited me recently for her routine three month checkup and asked, "How long will it take before I stop feeling so uncertain about life?"

I had to say, it depends. There is no "right" way to feel after cancer. The important thing is to handle your emotions in a way that works for you. Many survivors find it helps to talk their feelings out—with a close relative or friend, with other survivors in a support group, with a priest or rabbi, or even short term with a psychotherapist. Often a frank discussion with your doctor about what may be done to lessen the physical side effects of your treatment can also help you get through the initial feelings of isolation that separate you from the well world.

Fighting Fatigue

After treatment, many women discover that even the simplest task leaves them winded and tired, sometimes for weeks, even months after therapy. For some, energy levels never return to what they were before treatment. This fatigue can wreak havoc with fragile emotions. Frequently survivors complain: If I could just stop feeling so tired, I'd probably feel more positive about getting on with my life.

"When I get up in the morning, I'll make all these plans in my head to get tickets for the theater, or weed my front garden, maybe even hem those pants in my closet," says Mary, a fifty-year-old Californian who needed ostomy surgery and radiation for colon cancer last year. "But before I can even get out of bed, I feel this sense of exhaustion pass through me. I knew I might have trouble getting used to my physical scars, but I never envisioned that I would feel so drained and useless."

Cancer affects many of the day-to-day aspects of living, and when your energy is low, it can leave you wondering if your vitality for life will ever return. Here, the best advice is simple: Take your time. Feelings of exhaustion are warning signs that the body needs to rest, and the best response is to do just that. Getting yourself overtired can also fuel feelings of depression, not only weakening your physical defenses, but dampening your emotional spirits as well.

You shouldn't feel bad if you don't have as much energy as another survivor after treatment. Recovering from cancer is very, very individual and shouldn't be looked upon as a competition. You may feel drained and exhausted one week and the next week find you have more energy than you ever had because you're taking better care of yourself. Each survivor faces her own crises of emotions after treatment has ended. Some may have only short-term difficulties, while others endure major psychological problems that can be cured only by a combination of therapy and antidepressant medication.

When my own treatments ended, I made a mental note when my energy levels were highest and tried to schedule the bulk of my errands and activities during that time. It took about four months before my energy returned to optimum, and while it was frustrating not to be able to jump right back into life, I knew trying to do too much could also compromise my already depressed immune system.

The Power of Day-to-Day Living

During those first few months after treatment, you may find it hard to envision a time when cancer will not be your first thought when you awaken and your last thought before you fall asleep. But a time does come when cancer takes a backseat in your life, when the intense memories of therapy and the emotions surrounding it fade with time, and life can be enjoyed for its smaller pleasures.

After counseling patients over the last fifteen years, I can't help but note that the women who seem to do best are usually those who measure out their lives in day-to-day doses. As one psychologist put it: They learn to get up in the morning and pour the coffee, despite having had cancer.

Grace, a fifty-six-year-old widow who lost her larynx to throat cancer three years ago, was initially concerned that she'd never be able to read to her newborn granddaughter or, God forbid, scream out a warning should the youngster suddenly run away from her and into traffic. But after several months of working with a speech pathologist, Grace found she could speak and be understood without much problem.

"At first I was scared," she says, "but when I stopped looking too far into the future and focused instead on the day-to-day events in my life, things seemed more manageable.

"Now I follow my care plan, but I don't dwell on the disease or talk to others about it. Some I suppose well-meaning people at the office said that my reaction is called denial, and that it was bad for me. But I talked about it with my minister, and he said denial can be positive when it helps you get on with your life. I have my ups and downs like everybody else, but I feel good about the way I'm handling my disease."

During this period, it's important to take pleasure in the little markers of recovery. In the midst of my own ordeal with chemotherapy, my thumbnails and toenails turned black. Once treatment had ended, I remember the thrill of seeing the healthy nails begin to grow back, and I reveled in the chance to cut off even the slightest sliver of black. Each evening my husband would watch as I curled up on our bed, slowly snipping away at the grisly effects of my disease. For me, this was the final stigma, and clipping my nails became a symbolic gesture of casting aside the trauma of the past.

In some cases, however, the effects of treatment can be far more devastating, making it much harder—though not impossible—to find the smaller joys in life.

Jane and her husband, George, were anxiously expecting the birth of their first child. But when the time came for the thirty-eight-year-old kindergarten teacher to deliver, doctors discovered a massive tumor on one of her ovaries. In a surgery lasting five hours, Jane endured a cesarean section, the birth of her son, and the complete removal of her uterus, ovaries, omentum, and lymph nodes. A catheter was implanted in her abdomen to deliver chemotherapy directly to the site of her tumor. As a consequence, she developed a numbness and tingling in her fingers known as peripheral neuropathy. Moreover, the chemicals she received were so toxic that they caused a rare and potentially dangerous side effect called Lhermitte's sign.

Now, when she least expects it, a sudden and unexpected jolt of energy may race down her arm, sending a searing shock of pain through her hands. Fortunately Jane and George have developed a sort of gallows humor about these side effects: "I'm not so worried about her cooking in the kitchen as I am about her holding the baby," George told the oncologist recently with a chuckle. "Can you imagine if she were holding the baby and suddenly the shock ends up hurling him across the room. Wow, watch out. Human football!"

So that Jane can feed the baby a bottle, the couple have devised a sling that straps the baby across her chest. Chances are Jane's side effects won't last forever and she'll be able to regain full use of her hands. But until then, "I've learned to appreciate the life I still have, not what's lost," she says, grinning down at Michael, now fourteen months old. "It's been a long, uphill battle, but I'm not ready to call it quits yet," she adds. "Dealing with life after cancer has become like a job—some days you show up, even though you'd rather be at the beach. But you learn to give it your best shot, no matter what."

Survivors like Grace and Jane can teach others an important lesson: Once you've had cancer, you have to close the door and look straight ahead. Whether "straight ahead" turns out to mean two years left to life or twenty years and counting, life is a precious and magical gift to be lived in the fullest sense each and every day. Sure, there are darker moments when each woman loses self-confidence and begins to despair. But somehow these survivors have learned to take pleasure in the smaller, more common moments in life—not just the memorable occasions—and have found a sense of purpose and enjoyment to their lives no matter how long they last.

Attitude and the Immune System

Recently scientists have begun to investigate whether positive and negative emotions have an impact on the body's immune system. We know that patients who get cancer somehow have an impaired immune system. Otherwise they wouldn't get cancer in the first place. But as of yet no firm data exists to prove that positive thinking can bolster the body's ability to fight disease or, conversely, that negative thinking somehow limits or breaks down immune function.

I can say that through the years I've noticed anecdotally that my patients with a more positive attitude do seem to do better than those who have resigned themselves to die. Is it because there's something about the cancers that grow in certain patients that contributes to this attitude? We're still not certain.

Researchers have discovered a factor called cancer cachexia, which floats around in the blood of patients who have progressive disease. If, for example, you take blood serum from a patient who is about to die and inject it into yourself, you will feel that same cancer cachexia—the sense of literally wasting away—that characterizes many terminal patients. But do survivors with a bad attitude have a small measure of that substance in their blood, making it impossible for them to feel better? We don't know. Is there some natural component—perhaps endorphins in the brain—that augments the immune system and makes some survivors feel better than others? We don't know that, either.

When I first started as a oncologist, I had a patient who asked if I'd mind coming to the hospital to administer her chemotherapy a bit earlier each morning so she could make a seven A.M. tennis match. Down the hall from her lay another of my patients who had been totally bedridden from chemotherapy for almost six months. Interestingly, the one who was so full of zest and vigor ended up succumbing to her disease, while the woman who was so deathly ill from treatment has now survived for more than eleven years.

Granted, a positive attitude is important for coping with the challenges of this disease. But it doesn't alter the pathology of the tumor. As Harold Benjamin, director and founder of the Wellness Community in Santa Monica, California, so aptly points out: "There is life after cancer, life worth living, for those who want it, expect it, and work for it. . . . On the other hand, if you expect life to be miserable, it will probably be just that."

Reaching Out for Support

As you read this, I hope you don't take my message to be "Smile and get positive!" Getting cancer and living through treatment is a nightmare, a trauma that every woman has the *right* to feel terrible about and *needs* time to get over. No woman should be made to feel guilty over feeling sad and depressed for a while once treatment has ended. But sometimes the emotions can snowball into a more dangerous state of mind.

Six years ago, when she was thirty-nine, Sammie developed metastatic endometrial cancer. After chemotherapy and radiation, she suffered no further symptoms and today is, in all likelihood, fully cured of her disease. But as her oncologist, I practically had to hire a search team to drag her in for follow-up visits to make certain she was all right. "I'm fine, my husband's fine, my kids are fine. So why are you interfering with my life?" she said almost venomously after I'd managed to corral her into seeing me for a checkup.

I decided not to argue with her that day and examined her quickly, making a note to call her in six months. But several weeks later I got a call from Sammie's husband. In whispers he told me that he'd come home early from work and found his wife passed out on the couch, a bottle of bourbon by her side. At her last visit I'd noticed Sammie had gained weight and her face seemed a bit puffy. But now I knew for certain what I'd suspected to be true. Like some survivors, Sammie had begun drowning her fears and pain over cancer with alcohol and overeating.

Sally's story, though it lies at the other end of the emotional spectrum, is equally disturbing:

Seven years ago at fifty-one, Sally was one of the top interior decorators in Philadelphia, a veritable ball of energy who played tennis every morning, shopped the antiques dealers until five, and led an active life on the social circuit at night. But after learning she had ovarian cancer and submitting to seven months of chemotherapy treatments, Sally changed. She stopped playing tennis or visiting her friends. She closed her decorating business. And though free of cancer for the past six and a half years, she continues to have her husband drive her three and a half hours to New York and back—every two months!—so I can examine her for possible recurrence.

Though I've told her this is unnecessary, she still insists on having her blood tested each month for tumor markers of cancer. As she puts it: "Cancer is a black cloud that hovers over me every moment of every day. Everyone else seems to be in the sunlight, but it's always raining over me."

Lately her family has become angry and frustrated, insisting she get on with her life now that her health is normal. But she can't seem to get over the trauma of her illness and seems constantly to be waiting for the other shoe to drop.

Sad as it is to say, some survivors fall prey to severe bouts of mental illness despite a winning prognosis for good health. Often it occurs to women who have had a history of psychiatric disorders long *before* a cancer diagnosis has been made, says Jimmie Holland, M.D., chief of Psychiatry Services at Memorial Sloan-Kettering Cancer Center in New York. In addition, numerous studies on the psychological effects of cancer have shown that once treatment is over, the anniversary of the cancer diagnosis is frequently a trigger for clinical depression. In some cases survivors reexperience their diagnosis in nightmares and flashbacks so vivid that researchers have paralleled the reactions with those suffered by war veterans with post-traumatic stress syndrome. On the other hand, there is a phenomenon known as survivor's guilt, where patients begin to wonder why they've made it through to remission while others have not.

When Carol, a forty-two-year-old registered nurse from Seattle, discovered she had advanced ovarian cancer, doctors doubted she would survive her surgery, let alone ten months of experimental chemotherapy. Now, almost three years later, she is free of disease and planning to get married. But every time she visits her oncologist for follow-up, she feels a sense of overwhelming guilt.

"I can't help but look around at the other women seated in the waiting room who still have cancer," she says. "It makes me question why I'm doing so well, and I end up depressed. Most of the time I get on with my life just fine. But when I go to the doctor, the guilt eats at me for days afterward, and I feel like it's frustrating my progress."

The point here is, if you can't seem to shake the bad feelings you have about yourself, or if your anxieties seem overwhelming, get help! These days there are many options for getting emotional support, including cancer support groups and mental health professionals skilled in the specific issues and concerns of cancer survivors. Depending on the kind of care you need, a psychiatrist will be able to prescribe medication if problems such as severe depression and sleep disturbances become uncontrollable. Some specialists are also trained in hypnosis, behavioral modification, and relaxation techniques that can help reduce or relieve anxiety.

In chapter 10 I'll further discuss depression and stress and suggest ways to cope with these overpowering blockades that can dampen one's enjoyment of life. In the meantime, however, your doctor should be able to recommend a psychiatrist, psychologist, or social worker who can see you for short-term counseling.

Remember Gail, the spirited young lawyer with ovarian cancer who became so despondent she couldn't leave her home? A psychiatrist immediately placed her on antidepressant medication, and within six months Gail was back to her positive, vibrant, gutsy old self. As for Sally and Sammie, each could profit from psychiatric counseling to help them ventilate their anger and frustrations about getting cancer and help them reconcile their fears of recurrence.

To some degree, the threat of recurrence stalks every cancer survivor. Not knowing when and if cancer will reappear can sabotage the survivor's sense of mastery and control over her life. Like a sword poised to drop over Damocles' head, this fear can range from a general uneasiness about one's health to mild somatic complaints to pronounced anxiety or panic attacks that interfere with daily life. Not every survivor who worries about recurrence needs professional counseling. If you have a strong family support group and seem able to express your feelings and cope with the ups and downs of life, then you're probably doing fine. But if you see yourself in Sally or Sammie, Gail, or even Carol, it may be time to look outside your circle of family and friends for assistance.

Peer support may be another option to consider. Hundreds of survivors' groups are now active across the United States, providing support, advice, and practical assistance for survivors needing to talk about their problems and hear that they're not alone. Many groups meet regularly in private homes, hospitals, community houses, or places of worship. Other groups specific to the needs of a particular disability can provide an informal forum where survivors can share their concerns and get help in overcoming physical limitations caused by cancer. A list of support groups for survivors and their loved ones are contained in the "Resources" section that ends this book. If you can't find one in your area, ask your doctor or hospital social worker for recommendations.

But one final word of caution. Joining a survivors' group is a personal decision, and you shouldn't feel compelled to attend if it doesn't feel right. Every woman is different, and what works for one survivor may or may not work for you. Before you go, ask yourself if you're comfortable discussing your cancer with others and if you feel ready to hear the stories of others. If you attend and come out feeling depressed and anxious, give yourself some time before you consider visiting another peer group.

When my patients tell me they're looking for a survivors' group, I'm careful to tell them that there is always the chance some people in the group will die. That can be very disturbing to you as a survivor, especially if you've developed a bond with another woman who ends up not making it. It can shake your confidence and make you wonder whether you're truly a survivor or simply just holding on. More often than not, support groups are less concerned with disease and more with getting on with life. In them, you'll be able to address many of the emotional and physical hurdles you'll be tackling now that cancer is gone. But remember, while the battle to heal your body may be over, the fight to keep it happy and healthy has only just begun.

Tips for Coping During the First Few Months after Treatment

- *Be good to yourself.* Instead of trying to do everything for others, take some time off for yourself. Read a good book, have a manicure, take in a movie, or visit a new shop or art exhibit. Indulging yourself isn't selfish, it's good medicine for the mind.
- *Learn to say no.* You're in control of your life, and politely refusing to do something isn't rude, it's your right.
- *Pace yourself.* Not everything has to get done right away. If you're feeling overwhelmed, divide your list of tasks into manageable parts and prioritize them, being sure to delegate some of the work to others.
- *Take a walk.* It's the best kind of exercise to start with after treatment and will help clear your mind of tension and anxiety. Speak with your doctor about when you can resume normal activity.
- *Talk about your concerns.* Spoken out loud, worries have a way of seeming much smaller and less overwhelming. If you don't have a friend or family member to chat with, call your doctor and ask her advice.
- *Pick your battles.* Not every skirmish is worth winning, not every argument worth fighting over.
- *Look at the positive side.* Nothing in life is ever perfect, not even before cancer entered your life. So think about all you've achieved, and be proud of it.
- *Get enough sleep.* Feeling tired is your body's warning signal that it needs to rest and replenish its energies.
- *Laugh at yourself.* If your hair has just started to grow back, think of how goofy you look. If you can't raise your arm to get dressed in the morning, you may have a future as Quasimodo. When you're feel-

ing down, it's important to find something—no matter how self-deprecating—to giggle about and give yourself a lift.

- *Help someone else.* Whether it's picking up a quart of milk for the neighbor or testing your daughter for a geography test, reaching out to others can help you feel stronger and more in control of your own life.
- *Try something new.* Taking on new hobbies and learning new skills can bolster your self-image and make you feel better about your life that lies ahead.

Three

THE NEED FOR FOLLOW-UP CARE

Your treatment is now complete, your cancer in remission. Now, more than ever, you must be vigilant about your health and return to your doctor for regular follow-up exams. In most cases your oncologist or cancer surgeon will supervise your care, asking that you come in to be examined every two to three months the first year, every three to four months the second year, and every six months thereafter.

Because your well-being and good health are of chief concern, your doctor will use these visits to monitor for recurrence of cancer and examine you for delayed difficulties or potential side effects of surgery, chemotherapy, and/or hormonal or radiation treatments. Though these periodic checkups can serve to comfort and reassure some cancer survivors, most women find them a nerve-racking yet necessary ordeal.

"In the first couple of years after my recovery, the thing I hated most was going for my checkups," says Adele, a forty-two-year-old secretary from Brooklyn, New York. "Just seeing the hospital reminded me of a part of my life I'd rather have forgotten. I had almost a physical reaction to the sounds and smells of the place. But more than that, those visits reminded me that I'd been sick and that my cancer might recur. In my daily life, I'd kept those thoughts out of my mind. Fortunately it's better now. Maybe I've just gotten used to the routine. But I also understand how important these checkups are to my health."

Ingrid, a sixty-year-old housewife from Long Island, New York, found she had to allot an extra half an hour driving time before her visits, just in case she had to stop at a gas station to throw up. Another patient always asks her husband to come with her for each examination "so he can physically push me into the waiting room."

Standing in the patient's spot for a minute, I know how unsettling these initial few follow-up visits can be. When I first went to visit my own doctor after being treated for breast cancer, I felt as though I were sitting on a keg of dynamite. Every time he poked under my arms or examined my breasts, I was certain I'd explode. There were minutes of absolute terror while I waited for the results of my blood tests, then a feeling of sheer joy when everything looked normal. But the buildup, the anxiety, the waiting—at times it was excruciating. In fact, studies have shown that the fear of recurrence, along with the fear of the physician finding disease, can lead some survivors to develop symptoms of anticipatory nausea or hypochondria or even to avoid coming in for checkups altogether.

Nevertheless, the importance of follow-up care cannot be overestimated. As the numbers of cancer survivors grow, researchers are finding a disturbing array of long-term and late effects of therapies, making it all the more crucial for women to adhere to a regular schedule of follow-up cancer care.

Open communication with your oncologist is an integral part of survivorship. While the responsibility for it rests, in large measure, with your doctor, some of it is up to you. To help you better understand your care and make the most out of your regular checkups, here are some practical suggestions to follow.

Organize Your Thoughts

Before your first follow-up visit, sit down with a family member or friend and make a list of questions to ask your doctor. Write them down in a small notebook that you can carry in your purse, and jot down any concerns or issues as you think of them. Before each visit, look through your notes for any questions you may not have asked or concerns that you need better explained. Be sure to bring the notebook to the doctor's office and jot down any comments or instructions that seem important.

Draw up a list that includes *all* your symptoms—describing the obvious ones as well as any persistent aches or twinges you may be experiencing. Your doctor can't read your mind, so it's important to be frank. That means discussing any difficulties you may be having emotionally, any overindulgence in food or alcohol, any sexual problems, any pains or limitations you may be worried about. Be sure to note any medications you may be taking, including over-the-counter supplements like vitamins or laxatives. And find out if there are any nonprescription drugs you *shouldn't* take.

After finishing treatment for breast cancer, Margaret made a pact with herself to eat more nutritiously and take a daily calcium supplement to protect herself against osteoporosis and heart disease. But when she asked her druggist which dose of calcium she should be taking, he gave her a bottle of calcium with iron. After several weeks she began to develop severe stomachaches and grew frightened that her cancer had returned. Fortunately the problem was quickly resolved when her doctor discovered that the iron in her calcium supplements was to blame.

Based on your particular treatments and current state of health, your doctor will decide how often you need to be examined. It's a good idea to check how long each visit should take and whether you'll need to bring in urine or stool samples for testing. You'll also want to know whether there is a specific time each day that the doctor or her nurse can field simple questions over the phone and, in case of emergency, how to reach them in the evenings, on weekends, or over the holidays. Most likely your oncologist will take a vacation or periodically attend a medical meeting out of town, so you should ask who will be "covering" for him while he is away and whom to call in the event of a problem.

You'll also want a sense of the kind of diet you should be on. Depending on your cancer and the kinds of foods you like to eat, your doctor may advise you to limit your intake of fat and recommend a regimen of vitamins and supplements for good health. (In the next chapter I go into much greater detail about diet, nutrition, and lifestyle changes the cancer survivor should be making.)

Finally, make a note to ask your doctor how soon you can resume normal activities. If you've had recent surgery, you'll want to find out from your physician how quickly you can begin to exercise again, have sex, or go back to work. If you've developed physical limitations or side effects as a result of treatment, ask your doctor if there is a rehabilitation center or physical therapist you should contact. It's also advisable to check whether your immune system is strong enough to allow you to resume visits to the dentist or schedule any beauty treatments like a facial, manicure, or pedicure.

Stay Alert

At first it's hard not to react to every ache and pain as a sign of recurrent cancer. I tell my patients to make me a list and ask them to include even their slightest symptoms. More often than not, I end up reassuring them that it's nothing. But it helps when they write down their concerns, listing *all* the symptoms they may be worried about. Often, when they come in, they're a bit befuddled and intimidated to be seeing the doctor. Sometimes they'll forget what it was they wanted to discuss. If they bring me a list of complaints—no matter how minor they seem—I can go down it, point by point. I've looked at lists of symptoms half a page long and others ten pages in length. And I tell them the more complete the better. I'd much rather explain that a certain problem is common and nothing to worry about than risk missing something important.

"I find I walk a fine line between watching the way I should for signs of recurrence and going overboard," says Jill, a survivor of breast and uterine cancers. "I never used to be like this, but it's hard not to be scared by changes that might mean problems."

Knowing which signs of recurrence you should look for depends largely on the original site of your cancer. In survivors of breast cancer, for instance, we're particularly concerned about lumps that may have surfaced under the arms or in the neck, as well as any persistent bone pain, which could signal the spread of cancer into the lymph nodes or spine.

But every woman experiences an aching back, a stiff neck, or a headache now and then. If a certain symptom persists, get in touch with your doctor. Many patients confuse a variety of ills—the flu, menopause, arthritis, even the common cold—with signs of recurring cancer. However, pain is also your body's way of telling you something may be wrong, and for that reason you should never ignore it.

Between visits to your doctor, watch for any of the following problems:

- changes in your breast or in your scar area such as lumps, thickening, redness, or swelling
- pain in your breast, shoulder, hips, lower back, abdomen, or pelvis
- lumps in neck, under arms, in groin, or in breasts that could signal lymph node involvement
- persistent indigestion or gas
- nausea, vomiting, diarrhea, or heartburn that lasts for several days
- bloating or a feeling of fullness after a light meal
- irregular vaginal bleeding
- backache
- nagging cough or hoarseness
- fever
- loss of appetite or sudden, unexplained weight loss or gain
- dizziness, blurred vision, severe or frequent headaches, or trouble walking

Ask for Support

It's normal to feel anxious and worried about visiting your doctor for follow-up. Most women do. That's why many find it helps to bring along a tape recorder, or ask a friend or family member to come with them, to help them remember everything that's discussed. No matter how well you think you understand your case, it may be difficult to absorb everything the doctor will be telling you, especially if you're scared to hear what might be said.

If you feel uncomfortable or embarrassed to have a friend with you during your physical examination, ask your friend to take a seat in the waiting room. This way you can ask the doctor any particularly sensitive questions on your own, but still have someone there for support if needed.

What to Expect

During most follow-up visits, your physician will perform a complete physical examination. This exam will usually cover you from head to toes. Your physician is looking for swollen or enlarged lymph nodes, new lumps or masses, or swelling of your arms or legs. A pelvic examination is a crucial part of the checkup. If your oncologist is not performing a pelvic and rectal examination, ask for a referral to a gynecologist. This important examination should be done at least yearly and more often if you have had cancer of the breast, uterus, ovaries, cervix, vulva, or colon. Depending on where your cancer was diagnosed, you may also need all or some of the following procedures:

- a mammogram to screen for breast cancer
- blood tests to check for anemia, kidney and liver function, and other subtle changes
- tumor marker blood tests to check for heightened levels of cancer antigens
- a sonogram, CAT scan, and/or magnetic resonance imaging (MRI) to check for recurrence
- chest X-ray to check your lungs
- a bone scan to check for signs of recurrent cancer
- a Pap smear

- a sigmoidoscopy or colonoscopy
- a stool sample to screen for blood in the stool

Inform Your Doctor

To give you the best care possible, your doctor needs to have a sense about you as a survivor. The physical examination will give her some information, but only *you* can fill her in on how you're doing as a person. Start off by describing briefly what you've done that past week—whether it was taking in a baseball game, leaving work early, or arguing with your children. This will give her some clues to your emotional state of mind and help her know where to make suggestions about any difficulties you may be having. Be sure to discuss any changes in your lifestyle (good for you, you've stopped smoking!), which could warrant changes in the dosage of medication you may be taking.

It also helps to give your doctor an idea of how much you want—or don't want—to know about your cancer. Once their treatments are complete, many women make it their business to head straight to the library and track down stacks of information about their disease. But sometimes they misinterpret the facts in a particular medical article or news report. Staying up-to-date on your disease is important, and your doctor can help you figure out how the latest research pertains to you. On the other hand, some survivors prefer to put their cancer behind them and want to know as little about their case as possible.

"When I go to the doctor, I grit my teeth and put up with the examinations," says Edith, seventy-six, who had part of her bowel removed for colon cancer several months ago. "But I don't enjoy going, and frankly, at my age, the less I have to hear about my cancer, the better."

How much you understand your particular case will also depend on how well you understand your doctor. I confess that sometimes I'm just as guilty as the next oncologist of injecting too much medical jargon into my discussions. But as a patient, it's your right to be thoroughly informed about your health. So try to get the doctor to speak in simple terms, not medicalese, and have her explain why you'll be needing certain tests and what the results will mean.

Patty, forty-three, was diagnosed with such extensive ovarian cancer that I told her, rather than go in for a second-look surgery, we should go straight ahead and treat her with an additional series of chemotherapy. Soon, however, she developed severe side effects from the chemotherapy, so we had to stop. She began to develop pains in her abdomen, so we scheduled a CAT scan and sonogram. But before I had a chance to contact her with the results, she called my office, hysterical, screaming to my nurse that the tests showed a mass in her colon. When I looked at the X-ray report, the radiologist had written, "No sign of disease, faint activity in the upper abdomen and rectal region probably normal bowel decreasing with time." In plain English: gas! Instead of calling her oncologist for a translation and saving herself hours of anxiety and worry, Patty had misunderstood the medical jargon and panicked.

Remember: One of the problems with follow-up tests is that there are sometimes false-positive results, meaning there's an indication of a recurrence when actually none exists. These are the glitches and mistakes of modern medicine—no procedure is infallible. Before you assume the worst, your tests should be repeated. It's very rare for a physician to act on the basis of one test parameter.

Develop a Plan

To get a good picture of your individual needs, ask your doctor for a game plan of sorts: what you'll need to do this year—and in the future—to take care of your health. In addition to regular checkups, some survivors may need help in dealing with emotional or sexual problems, while others may seek pain control therapy, rehabilitation, or home care. Your doctor will be able to recommend a specialist skilled in your particular problem or limitation. In addition, she can help you find shopping sources for a prosthesis or any other medical products you may need.

After surgery for breast cancer, May Ling developed a frozen left shoulder, making it impossible to raise her left arm. For a violinist this was a disaster. But after practicing a set of physical therapy exercises for two weeks, she was able to move her arm freely.

"I still notice when I go into warm weather, I'll get this referred pain down my arm," she says. "But my doctor has explained that this usually occurs when surgery and radiation have been used together. She says a capsule of scar tissue has developed that traps and ends up injuring the nerves that run down my arm. Chances are it won't go away, but I've learned to live with it and still play the music I love."

If you've experienced any type of chronic pain since your treatment, make a note to inform your doctor. You may be able to take over-the-counter medications such as buffered aspirin, acetaminophen, or ibuprofen to relieve the pain. But first, before you take *any* medication, check with your doctor.

Stay in Contact

The other day I said to a patient of mine who'd had breast and ovarian cancer, "You know, you haven't gotten a mammogram in over a year." She'd been finished with treatment for many years, and most likely her cancers were cured. "You know," she answered, "some people get cancer and live with it on their mind all the time. They can't seem to shake the feeling. But I'm prepared to go on living despite my disease. I guess that's why the farther I get from my cancer, the more sporadic my visits. So I simply forgot about needing a mammogram."

As the months pass, and you distance yourself from the initial crisis of cancer and its treatment, you may find yourself reticent to continue follow-up care with your doctor. Though this is a natural response, only your oncologist knows the details of your treatment and the possibilities for long-term side effects.

One patient of mine named Roxanne had the lymph nodes under one arm removed as a consequence of breast cancer. One night she called my service to say she'd developed a painful infection in her thumb after clipping off a hangnail. I told her to go immediately to the emergency room, where she was treated for what could have developed into a life-threatening staph infection. Fortunately she was better in several days. But without her lymph nodes, her body's immune system was unable to fight off infection and disease, and she might have gotten quite sick without immediate intervention.

As time goes on, many women end up distancing themselves from their medical team, slipping into old routines and old habits. Although they remember the cancer experience as traumatic, the passage of time numbs their recall of events, giving them almost a selective memory of sorts. This can make staying in touch with one's doctor difficult, even downright annoying. But it's surely one of the best things a survivor can do to preserve her health and well-being.

Four

TAKING CARE OF YOUR HEALTH: DIET, NUTRITION, AND LIFESTYLE

*D*eep in the heart of every cancer survivor lies the nightmarish fear that one day the disease will return. That's why it's important to do whatever is possible to lessen that risk. Researchers now believe that cancer is the end product of a lifetime of insults to the body. While many of these so-called hits to the system are beyond our control—like our age, our genetic background, or whether we've gone through menopause or not—there are other risks we can lessen or eliminate to help protect ourselves against recurrence and future disease.

Evidence shows that losing weight and focusing on better nutrition and exercise may significantly decrease our chances of getting another cancer—even if we're at risk in other ways. Scientists now suspect that as much as 80 percent of all cancers may be related to environment and to things we eat, drink, and smoke. Though we cannot change where we live or do away with all the hidden chemicals in our environment that may contribute to cancer, it is within our power to make healthier lifestyle choices. That means choosing better foods to eat and exercising regularly, as well as giving up any bad habits like smoking or excessive use of alcohol—all of which experts now believe may well make the difference between promotion or prevention of the disease.

Every cancer survivor wants a clearer understanding of the factors that increase her odds against future disease. But many often find themselves confused and frustrated by much of the contradictory medical information and advice they hear about so regularly in the news. This chapter will help you sort through some of the mixed messages you've been receiving and bring you up-to-date with the latest scientific evidence on which foods and behaviors to avoid. It will also show you how a healthy lifestyle helps prevent disease and will give you some practical information to get started. You'll learn that you don't have to give up any of the foods you love or exercise like a maniac to protect yourself against cancer. Instead you'll see how some simple changes in diet and activity can work in your favor to deter the threat of cancer and help prevent heart disease, diabetes, and osteoporosis, which continue to strike millions of American women later in life.

How Too Much Fat May Promote Cancer

By now most survivors realize that cigarette smoking and unprotected exposure to the sun can cause cancer. But did you know that 60 percent of all cancers in women may be related to what they eat? Though experts are still not certain what dietary component causes cancer to develop, they suspect that fat may be one of the likely culprits.

Numerous studies show that eating too much fat (both saturated and unsaturated) may increase a woman's chances of getting cancers of the colon, breast, and endometrium. On the other hand, limiting the fat in your diet may reduce your cancer risk. A recent study for colon cancer found that women who get less than one-third of their calories from fat are 50 percent less likely to develop colorectal cancer than those who eat more fat.

Obesity is also a risk factor for cancer. Statistics show that overweight women have significantly higher rates of cancers of the endometrium, colon, and breast. Moreover, obese women run a much greater chance of breast cancer recurring and have a 55 percent higher risk of dying from it than those of normal weight.

Though researchers have yet to pinpoint how dietary fat promotes the growth of certain female cancers, they believe it touches off a complex chain of cellular and hormonal events that may trigger the disease and help existing tumors grow. Every woman secretes a hormone from the adrenal gland called androstenedione. As part of the body's normal metabolic function, this hormone is converted to a weak form of estrogen in the fat cells. The more fat you eat and the more weight you carry, the more fat cells you have and, in turn, the more estrogen builds up. Excess estrogen stimulates the development of uterine and breast tissue, which may cause some cancers to grow. In addition, some research indicates that a high-fat diet can end up suppressing the immune system, short-circuiting a woman's own natural ability to stave off disease.

Given the ominous role that fat may play in the onset of female cancers, it is imperative that survivors of these illnesses be especially careful to manage their weight and stick to a low-fat diet. Moreover, once a woman has had either uterine, breast, ovarian, or colon cancer, her risk of developing one of the other cancers is raised significantly. When I see these patients for their first post-treatment checkup, I tell them in no uncertain terms just how critical it is to drop any extra pounds and to limit their intake of fat. Last year a patient of mine named Marian was horrified when I handed her a two-cup measuring bowl and told her that was how much estrogen she'd been feeding into her body each day just by being overweight. Though her uterine cancer had been detected early, it had cost her her uterus. Unless the sixty-four-year-old homemaker made a concerted effort to lose fifty pounds, I said, she was almost certain to get breast or colon cancer. And next time she might not be so fortunate.

I also warn my patients that fat can interfere with the early detection of recurrent or secondary disease. When an oncologist performs a pelvic examination on a survivor who is overweight, she may be unable to differentiate the difference between fat in the abdominal region and any unusual swelling or lumps that signal the return of cancer. This is what happened when Connie, a forty-six-year-old schoolteacher, returned for her one-year follow-up for breast cancer, weighing in at 210 pounds. Though her pelvic exam seemed normal, I decided to get a vaginal sonogram of her pelvis. When the results came in, I was shocked. Deep inside her abdomen lay an ovarian tumor the size of a tennis ball. Fortunately for Connie, a hysterectomy and a bilateral salpingo-oophorectomy (removal of her uterus, tubes, and ovaries) was able to eradicate the cancer before it spread. But she now knows how important losing weight and staying on a low-fat diet are for good health and early detection of cancer.

The Controversy over Fat and Breast Cancer

The connection between fat and breast cancer still remains controversial. Although media headlines have recently dismissed any association between breast cancer and a high-fat diet, it's important to look a bit deeper at the facts behind the latest findings.

Last year, after analyzing the results of one of the largest and most respected studies on women's health, Harvard researchers found no link between dietary fat and the incidence of breast malignancies. Of the nearly 90,000 nurses who participated in the Nurses' Health Study since 1980, close to 1,500 developed breast cancer. But it didn't seem to matter whether they ate a diet as low as 25 percent fat or one as high as 44 percent: low-fat eaters still developed the disease, while high-fat consumers did not.

Even so, the study has been criticized because of the way its data was evaluated and because it selected a group of women—nurses—who may have already known what the "correct" answers were and recorded those rather than what they actually ate. Critics also contend that the women studied may not have been following a sufficiently low-fat diet.

Dr. Peter Greenwald, director of the National Cancer Institute's Division of Cancer Prevention and Control, believes that women may need to reduce the fat in their diets to 20 percent to truly lower their breast cancer risk. New research indicates that breast cancer patients who maintain such a low-fat diet actually *increase* their chances of a successful recovery, leading some doctors to theorize that cutting dietary fat is a feasible and potentially effective way to further reduce the risk of recurrence.

To find a definitive answer, the National Institutes of Health (as part of the Women's Health Initiative) has begun following several thousand women to see if cutting dietary fat by half can lower breast cancer rates. Unfortunately, results won't be in until the year 2006. In the meantime, most experts advise women who have had cancer to err on the side of caution and lower their intake of fat to 20 percent daily—both the saturated and unsaturated kinds.

The 20 Percent–Fat Solution

Some experts believe that if every American cut dietary fat intake to 10 percent daily, the risk of cancer would be cut dramatically. But let's be real. Unless you're the most disciplined, most determined woman in the world, a 10 percent–fat diet as a lifestyle is impractical, if not downright impossible. You would never be able to eat in a restaurant, go to a party, or have a piece of cake on your birthday. Before long you'd end up feeling so deprived and isolated that you'd rebel and probably go from a 10 percent–fat diet back up to a 50 percent–fat diet.

Instead, if you make sure that most servings of the foods you eat fall on or below the 20 percent mark each day, you'll be well on the road to healthier eating—and may lose a few unwanted pounds in the bargain. This way you can still indulge your cravings every so often, while getting the benefits of reduced cancer risk. No more than 10 percent of your total calories each day should come from saturated fats, with 6 to 8 percent as polyunsaturated fats and the remainder as monounsaturated fats.

These days the Food and Drug Administration requires that every food label display the total fat and saturated fat content per serving; some even list the percentage of fat in each portion. If they don't, you can do your own calculation. Since there are nine calories in a gram of fat, you'll need to figure as follows:

$$\frac{\text{grams of fat per serving} \times 9}{\text{total calories per serving}} = \text{\% of calories from fat}$$

For instance, let's take one serving of light sour cream (two tablespoons) that contains two grams of fat and thirty total calories according to the package label.

$$\frac{2 \text{ (grams of fat)} \times 9}{30 \text{ (total calories)}} = \frac{18}{30} = 60 \text{ \% !!}$$

Although two grams of fat does not seem like a lot, it's 60 percent of the total calories of this food product. When you're out grocery shopping, it's easy to be misled by "light" or "low fat" labeling. Check the labels carefully, and stay away from "health" foods such as granola cereal or "natural" fruit snacks. The term *natural* has no regulated definition when applied to snack foods, and they're usually packed with fat and sugar. Moreover, the claim "no cholesterol" does not mean "no fat," since vegetable oils (which do not contain cholesterol) can still be used.

When you're preparing a meal, be sure to calculate not only all the foods you'll be eating, but any oil or liquid they're cooked in. If you're dining out, this can be tricky. Try to order your food broiled or poached, without heavy sauces or dressings. Carry your own low-fat dressing in your purse, or use vinegar and olive oil sparingly, and order a decaf cappuccino for dessert instead of a more traditional high-fat treat. Once your palate adjusts to this healthier style of eating, you'll be surprised how simple and enjoyable it really is.

Tips to Cut the Fat

- Keep an honest food diary for two weeks. You will find out what (and how much) you eat. Identifying bad food habits is the first step toward changing them.

- Eat leaner cuts of meat, low-fat or no-fat dairy products, more seafood, and fewer fried foods.
- Trim all visible fat from meats before and after cooking; remove skin from poultry before cooking.
- Use nonstick pans for sautéing. Instead of oil, use chicken broth or spray lightly with vegetable oil.
- Use fruit preserves or unsweetened applesauce in baking instead of butter or margarine.
- Broil, grill, bake, poach, or steam your foods instead of pan-frying or deep-frying. Use a rack to allow fat to drip into a pan. Baste with wine, lemon juice, or orange juice. Do not use fatty drippings. Self-basting poultry can be high in saturated fat, so read the label first before you buy it.
- Instead of mayonnaise or sour cream, mix one third low-fat yogurt with two thirds low-fat cottage cheese. If possible, use a blender for the smoothest consistency.
- Substitute low-fat yogurt, skim milk, or buttermilk for cream in gravies and dressings. Yogurt will not separate when heated if you add one teaspoon of cornstarch per cup of yogurt.
- Use low-fat recipes. Look for cookbooks that list the calorie and percent of fat per serving in their recipes to help you eat the healthy way.
- Learn to use spice instead of fat to flavor your foods.
- Eat more fruits, vegetables, and whole grains. The National Cancer Institute and a number of other health organizations recommend that you eat at least five or more servings of fruits and vegetables a day to reduce the risk of developing colon and other cancers.
- Limit red meats and cheese. Instead use more poultry, fish, beans, and grains for sources of protein in your diet.
- Shop for low-fat or no-fat alternatives. You can still get the taste of high-fat dressings, dairy products, and snacks among the amazing variety of lowered-fat products on the market. Just be sure to read the labels carefully and beware hidden fat and sugar calories.

SWITCHING FROM HIGH-FAT FOODS TO LOW-FAT ALTERNATIVES

Instead of This	Try This
ice cream	nonfat frozen yogurt or sorbet
butter	unsweetened fruit preserves
cream soups	gaspacho, minestrone, consommé
sour cream dip	salsa
potato chips	pretzels
iced cake or doughnuts	angel food cake
brownies	gingersnaps, fig bars
croissants	plain bagel
salami, bologna	turkey, roasted lean ham
oil-packed tuna	water-packed tuna
french fries	roasted or baked potato
sour cream	yogurt or low-fat cottage cheese
corn chips	air-popped popcorn
cheddar cheese	part-skim mozzarella
one whole egg	one or two egg whites
ham-and-cheese omelet	vegetable-and-egg-white omelet
fruit-flavored yogurt	nonfat yogurt with sliced fresh fruit
olives	pickles
whole milk	skim milk

- Resist that second helping. Your brain needs twenty minutes to register that you are full.
- Don't try to be perfect. Your eating habits took a long time to develop and will take some time to change as well. If you try to cut

out everything, you'll end up feeling deprived and risk one high-fat binge after another. When you eat a high-fat meal, just try to balance it with low-fat foods the rest of the day. Keep low-fat, low-calorie nibbles on hand to cope with hunger pangs and cravings.

The Need for Fiber

When you switch to a low-fat diet, you may feel a bit deprived at first. In order to consume an adequate amount of calories each day, you'll need to increase your consumption of whole-grain and cereal products rather than relying on sugary foods to make you feel full. When sugar isn't used immediately by the body, it's converted straight to fat, and recent studies show sugar also may increase the incidence of colon and other cancers.

To lessen the risk of disease, the National Cancer Institute now recommends that all Americans double the amount of fiber they eat to between twenty and thirty grams daily—the equivalent of eating five half-cup servings of fruits and vegetables per day.

Fiber is the indigestible part of plant food, what some people still call roughage. Animal studies have shown that dietary fiber can reduce the risk of breast cancer, perhaps by influencing the body's metabolism of estrogen. Other research indicates that diets high in fiber may prevent colon cancer. While scientists still do not clearly understand how or which fiber-rich foods work best, they do know that certain types act like a scrub brush in the intestines, cleansing the bowel and helping the stool move out of the body more quickly. In doing so, fiber may help to counteract the dangerous effect of fat on the colon, say experts.

Among other things, fat digestion requires bile acids, which help the body absorb and use fat. The higher the fat content of the diet, the more bile acids may be released. Some of these bile acids travel from the small intestine, where fat absorption occurs, to the colon, or large intestine, where they are broken down by bacteria. Some experts believe that one of these breakdown products is the carcinogen 3-methylcholathrene, which may account in part for the association of colon cancer with a high-fat diet. But eating a high amount of fiber acts to bind with and remove bile acids, preventing potentially cancerous mutations in intestinal cells.

Fiber should be an important part of every woman's diet, particularly those who have survived cancer. However, fiber supplements are not the ideal choice. Instead, eat beans, whole grains, prunes, fruits, and vegetables like cabbage, corn, broccoli, carrots, and peas. Researchers still cannot state clearly whether the anticancer benefits of these foods come from their fibrous content, their vitamins, or both. Nevertheless, fiber does promote bowel regularity, which can be helpful for women who may have problems with constipation following chemotherapy or radiation to the abdomen or pelvic area. It also helps prevent intestinal problems such as diverticulosis (abnormal pouchlike sacs in the colon), which can result from chronic constipation or poor bowel habits. And because fiber-rich foods are bulky, giving you a satiated feeling, they can even help you control your weight.

It takes a concerted effort to assure there are *five* fruits and vegetables in your diet each day. Here's the strategy I find works best for me: a glass of orange juice and a fruit for breakfast; a huge salad of greens, mixed vegetables, and a pasta for lunch; a fruit or box of raisins midafternoon; and a salad or vegetable with fish at dinner. Other survivors try to chomp on carrots throughout the day, eat dried fruits for snacks, or have a baked apple or fruit salad for dessert, doing whatever it takes to get as much fiber as possible into their diets.

To gauge their success, I generally ask my patients, "How does your stool look?" This may sound like a disgustingly personal question, but often it helps me assess just how much fiber or fat a woman is eating. When an individual's stool is excreted in small, marblelike balls, it generally means that semisolid waste is staying too long in the colon. If the stool is excreted in one long column, then enough fiber is being eaten. Next I ask, "Does your stool float? Does it rise to the top of the waterline?" Your stool should sink to the bottom of the toilet; if it doesn't, you're eating too much fat.

Some women with colostomies may have to add fiber tablets to their diet, while people with ileostomies or who have had pelvic radiation may not tolerate fiber well. Speak to your oncologist to see what your individual needs are for good nutrition. And be sure your fiber-rich diet includes plenty of liquids to prevent dehydration.

Limit Your Protein

For some time, medical experts have known that the consumption of large amounts of protein may be associated with cancers of the breast, uterus, kidney, colon, pancreas, and prostate. Evidence shows that when protein reaches the colon, it is fermented by certain bacteria, which in turn releases certain carcinogenic substances. When you eat complex carbohydrates, you decrease the level of this protein fermentation.

All of us need a certain amount of protein in our diets to maintain good health. But to stay safe, many doctors now advise cancer survivors to limit the amount of animal protein in their diet to four ounces daily or to eat vegetable sources of protein like beans and rice or soy products like tofu or tempeh.

Drink Alcohol Rarely, If at All

Alcohol is a known risk factor for cancer. Since some studies have shown that moderate to heavy drinkers have a higher rate of breast cancer than nondrinkers, cancer survivors should be cautious and are advised to drink limited amounts, if at all.

An early report from an ongoing five-year study of sixteen thousand women at Harvard University and the University of Wisconsin now shows that women who consume two drinks a day have a 50 percent increase in breast cancer risk compared with nondrinkers; having three or more drinks doubles the risk. In addition, age appears to be especially crucial: regular drinking before thirty poses the highest overall risk, according to one study published in the *Journal of the National Cancer Institute*. Another recent study showed that women who began drinking later in life had higher than normal rates of breast cancer, suggesting that alcohol may act as a cancer promoter rather than as an initiating factor. Alcohol also appears to impair the body's ability to metabolize folate—a B vitamin that has been shown to reduce the risk of colon cancer.

The combination of alcohol and tobacco is especially deadly. Alcohol seems to work with tobacco to intensify cancer risk many times. Recent studies indicate that heavy drinking, particularly when combined with cigarette smoking, significantly increases your risk of cancers of the mouth, throat, esophagus, bladder, and liver.

Also remember that alcohol is a source of empty calories. It increases the appetite and contributes to obesity. If you continue to use alcohol because of its so-called benefits to the heart, take heed. While studies have shown that moderate amounts of alcohol seem to raise high-density lipoprotein (HDL) levels that may limit the buildup of arterial plaque, too much alcohol can raise your risks for breast cancer and liver disease. If you're going through menopause, it can also make hot flashes worse. If you have to drink alcohol at all, the American Medical Association recommends a maximum of one to two ounces a day—the equivalent of one or two glasses of wine or a shot of hard liquor.

The Caffeine-Cancer Conundrum

There still is no definitive proof that caffeine—either in coffee, colas, or chocolate foods—causes cancer. Nevertheless, widespread interest in this issue prompted the World Health Organization to commission a panel of experts to review the reams of data examining the effect of caffeine and coffee on the risk of cancer. In 1991 the panel found inadequate evidence that coffee or caffeine causes cancer of the breast or of the pancreas and other organs. Nor does coffee increase the risk of benign breast lumps, as was once believed. However, the consensus panel felt that there may be a link between bladder cancer and caffeine.

More recently, coffee's effect on pancreatic and bladder cancer was studied again. Ironically, coffee drinkers were shown to have a lower risk of pancreatic cancer than nondrinkers. Moreover, scientists from Yale University have found that twenty years of research on coffee and bladder cancer yielded no association between the two.

Even so, some doctors—including my own—feel it's important for cancer survivors to decrease their consumption of coffee, both the caffeinated *and* decaffeinated varieties. In my own effort to err on the side of caution, I've made an attempt to limit my intake of coffee to two cups of decaf a day. Maybe this will have no effect whatsoever on whether I ever develop cancer again. But given the alternative, I'm willing to give it a try.

What About Supplements?

Over the past decade, there has been increasing scientific and public interest in the possibility that certain vitamins, such as beta-carotene (vitamin A), vitamin E, and vitamin C, may help prevent cancer. It has been suggested that these micronutrients might have the ability to correct the damage caused by oxidation in the cells.

Eager to announce a magic pill to prevent cancer, the media has jumped on the bandwagon to promote the antioxidant effects of these vitamins, despite the fact that long-term studies to fully test the potential benefits—or hazards—of taking antioxidant vitamins have yet to be performed. The scientific community agrees there is still too much confounding data to recommend taking these vitamins as supplements. Nevertheless, exaggerated health claims abound in health food stores, on talk shows, and throughout the media for the taking of these so-called anticancer vitamins.

Last year, in a surprising and unexpected turn of events, the National Cancer Institute released the results of a major study that showed that vitamin supplements have no protective benefit on cancer *or* heart disease. Nevertheless, experts involved in the research said that the advice to eat lots of fruits and vegetables still stands, since the benefits found in earlier studies may have come from something in the foods other than vitamins.

With few exceptions, nature doesn't package a single cancer-preventing nutrient in a particular food. That's why it's important not only to moderate your intake of fatty, unhealthful foods, but also to balance your diet with a *variety* of fruits and vegetables. Evidence shows that cruciferous vegetables like broccoli and cabbage may reduce your risk of colon cancer, while foods rich in beta-carotene like carrots and winter squash may limit your risk for bladder, lung, and cervical cancer.

But too much of any one food may not be wise, either. Take the intriguing case of Dorit, a fifty-eight-year-old Israeli woman who decided several years ago to eat large numbers of foods with beta-carotene after several of her close friends developed breast cancer. Though her vegetarian diet was extremely healthy to start with, she began consuming huge quantities of butternut squash and carrots each day, all but eliminating any leafy vegetables and fruit from her diet. All seemed fine until a routine checkup revealed a small but suspicious mass in her pelvis. After three hours of surgery, Dorit required a hysterectomy and removal of her ovaries for an early ovarian cancer, but no further treatment. Still, her oncologist was perplexed; during surgery he'd noticed that most of her internal organs had a peculiar orange-yellow tinge. After giving her the good news that cancer had been caught early, he questioned Dorit about her diet, soon discovering that his patient had developed the rare but certain signs of beta-carotosis—an overdose of beta-carotene.

By changing her diet to emphasize one particular nutrient, Dorit may have missed the cancer-preventing qualities of other essential nutrients; this may have interfered with her body's natural ability to stem the growth of cancer. Though it is impossible to know for certain, Dorit now prescribes to a balanced and varied diet, with five or six *different* fruits and vegetables per day.

Doctors also recommend against taking "megadoses" of antioxidant vitamins to help protect against cancer. Until researchers can disentangle the positive effects of vitamins from those of other compounds found in foods, it's best to eat the whole food and not any refined portion of it. Overdoses of some vitamins, even small excesses, can produce harmful or toxic conditions.

The Need for Calcium

Because few women consume adequate amounts of calcium in their diets, most experts recommend calcium supplements. Early research indicates that taking calcium may reduce the risk of colon cancer. Moreover, various studies have shown that calcium supplementation can help to prevent deterioration in bones that leads to osteoporosis in older age. However, calcium supplementation alone cannot totally protect against osteoporosis—one needs to add exercise with or without hormonal replacement therapy.

The recommended daily allowance (RDA) of calcium for premenopausal (nonpregnant) women is 800 milligrams daily; women over fifty need 1,500 milligrams per day (1,000 if they are taking estrogen). It is best to begin taking extra calcium in your thirties.

Though calcium carbonate is the most popular supplement (found in Tums, for example), it generally is poorly absorbed by the body. Better to take 1,500 milligrams of calcium citrate over the course of a day—500 milligrams at each meal, for instance. Your calcium pill must dissolve quickly in the stomach to be absorbed. You can check your brand by placing it in white vinegar (which is acid, like stomach juices); it should dissolve in thirty minutes. If your dairy intake is low, or you live in a northern climate subject to long periods without sunshine, nutritionists also advise taking 400 IU of vitamin D daily, to help your body's absorption of calcium.

But first check with your doctor. You may be eating enough calcium-rich foods like dairy products, broccoli, soybeans, and green leafy vegetables to warrant a lesser dose of calcium each day. Keep in mind, too, that both caffeine and alcohol increase the loss of calcium through your stool and urine—another good reason to limit, if not eliminate, them from your diet.

The Need for Exercise

To reap the full health benefits of a low-fat, high-fiber diet, it's important to add regular physical activity. When women get older, their metabolism slows down, causing them to put on extra pounds. That's why many of my patients complain that while they are strict and conscientious about what they eat, their weight continues to climb. In addition, when women go into menopause, either naturally or because of cancer treatment, the levels of hormones in their body change, exacerbating any weight problem they already may have. As a consequence, many women find they must not only decrease what they're eating, but also increase their activity to maintain their weight. My patients will complain that while they are eating less and exercising more, their weight stays the same. That's because their metabolism has slowed down with age.

On the other hand, if a woman continues to overeat and has a sedentary lifestyle, she may soon find herself well on her way to obesity and at dangerous risk for recurrence or secondary cancers. Several studies suggest that breast cancer risk is lower among female athletes and among women who have engaged in moderate physical activity. In addition, exercise appears to have a modest effect on the development of cancer of the colon and pancreas. Some researchers have even shown that aerobic exercise can stimulate the immune system to produce antibodies and natural killer cells that destroy viruses, perhaps even cancer. Equally important, regular exercise can help you reduce your risk for chronic diseases and degenerative conditions like coronary heart disease, diabetes, osteoarthritis, and osteoporosis.

Last winter, when a patient of mine named Rosalie had a hysterectomy for uterine cancer at the age of fifty-six, she decided she finally had to do something about the extra twenty-five pounds she'd been carrying for years since the birth of her three children. She joined an aerobic step class at her local YMCA, and within six months she had lost nearly eighteen pounds. "At first I felt like a klutz. My arms would go one way and the rest of the class would go the other way. But laughing at myself felt good, and having that hour to myself three times a week became a luxury I never want to give up. Now I've developed a group of friends at the club, and I look forward to going. It's as if getting cancer gave me a new lease on life."

For another patient named Luisa, exercise provided an even wider range of benefits. Two days after her first granddaughter was born, Luisa lost her left breast to cancer. Soon after surgery she began a series of gentle upper-body exercises to help her regain normal movement of her arm. "It was stiff and painful at first, but I knew if I wanted to hold the baby, I had to stick with it," says Luisa, who admits she never exercised a minute before her cancer. Within several weeks, however, the Cuban-born homemaker was able to lift her infant granddaughter from her crib, cradle her while she fixed a bottle, and even hoist her up in the air to make her smile. "Now I've started to walk for a half hour each morning with one of my neighbors," adds Luisa, proud of her new accomplishments. "At first it was a way to keep my mind off the cancer, but now I look on it as practice for keeping up with the little one when she learns to walk."

Women like Rosalie and Luisa are disproving the common myth that once you hit middle age, it's too late to benefit from exercise. Most women over fifty were raised to believe that exercise was what men did, and that it wasn't considered a female responsibility to be athletic. But once you've been diagnosed with cancer, age is no longer the issue. Staying healthy is what counts.

Starting a Fitness Program

Before you begin any exercise program, you should consult with your doctor. Each woman has individual needs and limitations. You need to know what yours are, and you need to respect them. Some forms of radiation or chemotherapy have the side effects of weakening the heart muscle or diminishing lung capacity, precluding some survivors from certain types of exercise. Other survivors suffer from peripheral neuropathy (a numbness and tingling in the feet and hands) that may warrant a special type of footwear or exercise program to minimize accidents. Moreover, if you are obese or have other underlying health problems, your doctor may refer you to a supervised exercise program where you can be monitored more closely.

But no matter what your condition, it's important to start gradually and not overdo it. To get a modest, disease-preventing dose of exercise, you don't have to wind yourself or work out until your bones creak and your muscles are sore. Many survivors start with twenty minutes of fast walking, biking, or jazz dancing, two or three times a week, because they're vigorous enough to burn calories and interesting and moderate enough to keep doing them on a regular basis. Over the next few weeks, as your stamina increases and your legs get into shape, you'll find it easier to increase your pace and the amount of time you exercise, eventually building to a one-hour workout several times a week.

The best exercise is one that you'll keep doing. If you find yourself lonely or frightened to walk alone, find a partner or a health club with an indoor track. If your temperament leans more toward group activities, but you're unsure of your stamina, try a water aerobics class at a local pool or evening dance class at a local high school. If you find yourself getting bored with a particular exercise routine, switch to something else. It's a lifetime of activity that counts, not a surge of exercise one week and nothing the next. So choose exercise that you like, and vary the activity to keep yourself interested.

Biking, hiking, skiing (especially cross-country), aerobic dance, or speed walking are all wonderful fitness activities. Other sports like tennis or racquetball may seem strenuous enough, but if you're taking frequent rest periods within the game, you may not be getting enough *steady* activity. Golf is a poor exercise for conditioning, say experts, unless it includes rapid, prolonged walking. In addition to walking, swimming is an ideal program of exercise, especially if you've had minor orthopedic problems or arthritis. Because of its low impact and low risk of fractures, swimming is not particularly suited for older women with osteoporosis, because it is not weight bearing and has no effect on bone density.

If you find poor weather is hampering your determination, you might try one of the many indoor exercise machines on the market. Stationary bicycles or treadmills have been used for years in rehabilitation programs and are perfect alternatives when inclement weather keeps you stuck indoors. To overcome the boredom of pedaling to nowhere, many women watch television, read a book, or listen to music during their workout.

Exercise should feel pleasantly tiring. If it is just pleasant, you are probably not working hard enough; if it is only tiring, you are working too hard. As you slowly increase your level of endurance with each session, try using the "sing-talk method" to measure how hard you're working out. If you cannot talk without gasping for breath while exercising, you're probably working too hard; if you can sing while exercising, you're probably not pushing hard enough. Your objective for the first few months should be to stay injury free and healthy and then set up a routine that becomes a lifelong habit.

No One Is Perfect

Implementing your decision to change your eating habits isn't always easy. Nor is finding the time and the motivation to stick to a regular exercise program. Though most survivors want to take a healthier stance in their lives, many complain that the demands of work and family life seem to sabotage their good intentions. "I have two teenage sons and a husband who are constantly bringing high-fat treats and snacks into the house," said Clara, a forty-three-year-old breast cancer survivor. "As hard as I try to shop for healthy alternatives, the ice cream is always in the freezer at night, beckoning me to eat it."

In another example, Patricia, a fifty-five-year-old uterine cancer survivor, found it next to impossible to lose weight after surgery "because my husband always insisted on taking me out to dinner with friends to celebrate my getting past cancer."

Making a lifetime commitment to any program—be it diet *or* exercise—is never simple. Before my own ordeal with cancer, I used to pride myself on being the only woman in her forties who hadn't watched a Jane Fonda tape. Like many doctors, I'd learned to subsist on coffee, nervous energy, and whatever looked good in the hospital's snack machines. My eating habits were atrocious and my lack of exercise even worse.

But after cancer and its treatments were finished, I realized I had to adopt a healthier lifestyle or there wasn't going to be any of me left. So I began by switching to a fish and vegetarian diet, coupled with a weekend program of speed walking. Though it took me several months, I've gradually built up to an hour every Saturday and Sunday morning. I can't say I always look forward to it or that I enjoy putting aside precious time that I need for other things. No one does. But when I'm finished and return home tired but exhilarated, I realize how important my efforts really are to stay healthy and cancer-free.

Still, the farther you get from your cancer treatments, the easier it is to slip up. Instead of getting up one morning to exercise, you put it off for later that day, forgetting you have other commitments. Or maybe you grab a pastry at the local deli on the way to work or a box of buttered popcorn at the movies for a late night snack. Before you know it you've gobbled down a couple of thousand calories and more than a week's worth of fat.

In today's society fatty food is everywhere and there's always a good reason not to exercise. As a consequence, it takes a fair amount of discipline and advanced thinking to make smart choices, as well as the ongoing support of your family and friends to succeed.

Susan, a nurse and mother of two small children, vowed that after her chemotherapy for breast cancer was over, she'd make more of an effort to eat right and get regular exercise. "But somehow the days seemed to slip through my fingers," she recalls. "If I wasn't cleaning up after the kids or picking up the dry cleaning, I was at the hospital caring for patients, grabbing a quick meal in the cafeteria between shifts. By the end of the day I'd slip into bed feeling guilty and beat, worried that cancer would one day get the better of me again."

Her husband, an occupational therapist, was concerned as well. So one night after the kids were asleep, he led Susan to the couch for a chat. "I don't care if the dirty dishes are left in the sink or the beds are not always made," he told her, stroking her hand. "What I care about most is having you here by my side."

Together they decided on a plan that would let Susan take the time she deserved for herself. They'd each get up a half hour earlier in the morning, letting Susan begin a daily walking program while he watched the kids and fixed her a healthy brown bag lunch she could take to work.

"Just knowing that he cared and was willing to help made me realize that taking time for myself was worth the trouble," says Susan. "Now, when I feel guilty about leaving a mess, I remember that little chat and it reminds me that I owe it to my family as well as myself to stay healthy."

Helpful Strategies

After chemotherapy for ovarian cancer, Margarite found her taste buds were shot. "The only thing I could taste were sweets," she recalls. "After every round of treatment, I'd head for the malt shop and order a chocolate milkshake. It staved my thirst and got the metallic taste of chemotherapy out of my mouth, and it was my reward for getting through another round of treatment." But once her therapy was finished, the lawyer continued to succumb to her cravings, eventually gaining fifteen pounds before her three-month checkup at the oncologist's office.

These quirky desires for particular foods are common among cancer survivors. Some researchers believe high-fat/high-sugar foods, like chocolate and ice cream, actually have a relaxing effect on the body by causing endorphins—the body's natural painkillers—to be released in the brain. New research out of Rockefeller University in

New York City suggests that higher levels of certain brain chemicals may confer a "fat tooth," enhancing one's appetite for high-fat foods. If this theory is true, scientists may one day develop medications to help control these cravings.

However, until that happens, the two best ways to deal with cravings are either through distraction or confrontation. In the distraction approach, you need to find ways to ignore the urge to eat. Force yourself to think about every activity you've done throughout the day, plan what you want to get accomplished tomorrow, call a friend, or walk out the front door and down to your mailbox and back—anything to take your attention away from food. You'll have to distract yourself only for a few moments, because cravings generally pass within minutes or even seconds.

If you find yourself bombarded by a hankering for a certain food, confront your urges. For instance, before you stop at the ice-cream stand, pull over and take a minute to analyze why you want a treat so badly. Are you tired? Hungry? Feeling lonely or deprived? Now that you recognize what's propelling you toward the wrong food, set your mind not to let it get the best of you. Tell yourself: I'm in charge of my life and my weight. If I can get through having cancer, I can get through a few minutes of cravings. I'm the boss here, not some gloppy, disgusting ice-cream cone! Now drive home, and be proud of yourself. Chances are you'll face down your craving and end up overcoming the urge.

Inevitably, however, there will be times when willpower fails us. Last week all I could think about was a Reese's peanut butter cup. And by the weekend I ended up giving in. Let's face it, we're all human. And having an occasional treat is fine, as long as it doesn't turn into a steady diet. To stay sane and healthy at the same time, it's best to make some dietary trade-offs and plan for your favorite treats. If you know you have a special dinner party at the end of the week, try to be stricter with yourself in the days before. That way when you indulge in that slice of key lime pie, you won't feel so guilty.

Many survivors have developed strategies to help them through those hurried moments of their day when good eating habits have a way of getting forgotten. One of my patients is an advertising director who finds herself constantly on the run. In the morning before work, she packs her purse with a snack pack of raisins, cut-up carrots, Healthy Choice no-fat cheese sticks, and a can of soda water. That way, if she's stuck on an airplane or in a meeting, she doesn't have to resort to high-fat fast food to satisfy her cravings.

Changing your eating habits for the better does require a bit of planning. Inventory your eating habits and the items in your pantry. Throw away any foods that are high in fat and start keeping a journal of your eating habits to see which times of day you're most vulnerable to cravings and what kinds of stress drive you to eat. Review your diary every week to see what high-fat foods you eat, then seek out low- or no-fat alternatives. You don't have to eliminate the foods you love. Just choose *more often* the foods that help reduce your risks of cancer and choose *less often* the foods that might increase your risks.

You'll also need to be especially cautious at the supermarket. Even though new food-labeling laws have forced manufacturers to get honest about the dietary content of their foods, there still may be calories where you least suspect them. While a food may be accurately labeled low-fat, it still may be laden in starch, fructose, and diglycerides (which do not count as fat on food labels), making it dangerously high in calories. Keep in mind that when calories aren't burned by the body, they're converted into fat. That's why measuring the quantity of food you eat is just as important as monitoring its fat content.

Moreover, don't take every health-conscious claim at face value. In 1991, when McDonald's and Burger King stopped cooking their french fries in animal fat and switched to vegetable oil, they were widely praised for taking a big step in the right direction. But recently, University of Maryland researchers have discovered that foods cooked in vegetable oil have eight times more trans-fatty acids than foods cooked in animal fat. Trans-fatty acids, though technically unsaturated, *act* like saturated fats, raising blood cholesterol levels. In practical terms, whether cooked in animal fat or vegetable fat, fast-food fries never will be examples of healthy eating. They're just too high in fat, period.

Finally, be realistic. It takes time to break old habits. It helps to eat on a regular schedule so your blood sugar doesn't drop too low and drive you toward a binge. If you do have a setback, it's not the end of the world. Just chalk it up to learning a new lifestyle and move forward. If you make a promise to exercise three times a week but can't live up to it, set aside an extra half hour on the weekend. If, after a month, you still have trouble sticking with your diet or exercise program, ask your doctor for guidance. Many survivors consult with a registered dietitian or exercise counselor for personalized advice and healthful support.

Other Threats

A healthier lifestyle means more than just eating right and getting regular exercise. To really cut your risks, you have to give up any remaining bad behaviors, like excessive use of alcohol or smoking.

Smoking

If you're a cancer survivor and still continue to smoke, you might as well put a gun to your head and fire: sooner or later it will kill you. Evidence shows that tobacco eventually kills close to 25 percent of those who use it. And over four hundred thousand Americans die each year from tobacco-induced diseases, including cancers of the lung, head and neck, esophagus, bladder, pancreas, and cervix. New research also shows that smokers show increased risk for leukemia, a disease that previously has had few known preventable risk factors.

Although past research has indicated that cigarette smoking may actually protect against the development of breast cancer, a new report by the American Cancer Society shows that a woman's risk of dying from breast cancer *increases* by 25 percent if she is a smoker—and rises in proportion to the number of cigarettes smoked per day and the total number of years smoked. Other studies have shown that smoking also can have deleterious effects on the immune system, which could contribute to the poorer prognosis among breast cancer survivors who smoke.

If you have put off quitting for fear of gaining weight, you don't have any more excuses. New research shows that weight gain after quitting is usually modest and temporary—generally no more than five pounds gained.

But to kick the habit and make it stick, experts advise smokers to get a coach. Whether it's a committed listener, a self-help group, or a behavior modification expert, find someone who will keep you focused on breaking the habit and recommitting to good health every day.

The new nicotine patches can help, but they seem to work best in conjunction with a behavior modification support group. Recently one of my patients asked me for a nicotine patch to help her quit smoking. She had just delivered a baby, and I was treating her for an abnormal Pap smear—a condition related directly to smoking. I wrote out a prescription for the nicotine patch and advised her that she needed to join a smoking cessation group. But she neglected to tell me she was still nursing. When she got home and read the package insert, she called me, very upset. How could she stop smoking now and expose her baby to the nicotine from the patch? I was amazed she had no idea that nicotine and other cancer-promoting substances had been transmitted to her baby by smoking throughout her pregnancy and now while nursing. I advised her that the patch would actually be less harmful than the cigarettes, but that she certainly could quit without it, provided she had the support of a trained therapist or smoking cessation group.

Unprotected Sun Exposure

Soaking up the sun is one of life's greatest pleasures. But these days getting a tan isn't healthy, it's downright dangerous. A history of sunburns and a family background are the two main risk factors for malignant melanoma, a deadly form of skin cancer that strikes thousands of women each year. Though curable if detected early, it can spread like wildfire if not treated promptly, attacking other organs of the body via the bloodstream or lymphatic system. While the more common skin cancers known as basal and squamous cell carcinomas are usually slower growing, they can invade nearby areas and, in rare cases, spread to other parts of the body if diagnosed too late.

Skin cancer is the most common form of cancer in the United States. By the year 2000 it is expected that one in every seventy-five Americans will develop melanoma and one in seven will have some form of skin cancer. The disease, say dermatologists, is an undeclared epidemic.

Unprotected exposure increases the risk of skin cancer by damaging immune system cells in the skin. The best means of preventing it is through the use of sunscreens or sunblocks with an SPF (sun protection factor) of at least fifteen, applied thirty minutes before going outdoors and reapplied often, especially after swimming. It is also wise to keep your time in the sun to a minimum, regardless of the time of day or year. If you go to the beach, bring a parasol or beach umbrella; also, cover your arms with a long-sleeved T-shirt and wear a large-brimmed hat.

Regular self-examinations are an important part of early detection. Examine your skin every three months. Most skin moles are harmless, but as you look over any moles, birthmarks, or brownish areas, be sure to ask yourself these questions: Has it changed in size, thickness, shape, or texture since you last saw it? Does it have an irregular border? Is it bigger than a pencil eraser? If you find a new mole, is it translucent, tan, brown, black, or multicolored? If you answer yes to any of these questions, notify your oncologist. You should also call your doctor if you have a sore that is itchy or painful, bleeds continually, or does not heal within several weeks.

Food Additives and Meal Preparation

There is no good evidence that other elements of the American diet—food additives, pesticides, irradiated vegetables, or artificial sweeteners—play a role in the development of human cancers. In fact, some preservatives actually may protect against cancer.

However, some cooking methods—such as high-temperature grilling, smoking, salt curing, and pickling—can produce possible cancer-causing substances in foods. Research shows that these foods appear to increase cancer risk in people who eat them regularly and in large amounts. Occasional charcoal grilling, for example, does not appear significantly to increase cancer risk, although it is wise to avoid eating charred foods. And while it is safe for most people to eat smoked or pickled fish in moderation, if you smoke or have a history of stomach cancer in your background, it may be wise to avoid them.

Certain high-temperature food preparations like microwaving and boiling of vegetables and fruits also may destroy the cancer-protective qualities of these foods. Better to steam them lightly for three to four minutes or enjoy eating them raw in a salad or crudite.

HOW TO AVOID THE PITFALLS OF RESTAURANT EATING

- Don't be shy about asking how a certain dish is prepared before ordering.
- Avoid cream-based soups and any deep-fried or breaded foods.
- Ask that poultry or fish *not* be basted with butter or fat during cooking. If that's not possible, simply don't order it.
- At salad bars, skip the mayonnaise-type salads like coleslaw, tuna, and macaroni dishes. They're laden with fat.
- Ask for a double-size salad instead of roasted, whipped, or fried potatoes.
- Avoid dishes made with a lot of cheese, such as veal parmigiana, quiche Lorraine, and some Mexican dishes.
- If you're ordering Chinese food, stay away from the fried appetizers and main courses with a lot of sauce. Instead, order stir-fried vegetables and plain rice.

A WORD ABOUT ALTERNATIVE CANCER REGIMENS

After fifteen years of treating thousands of women for cancer, I find that I am often called upon to field questions about the myriad alternative anticancer regimens available today. Shark cartilage, raw juice therapy, shiitake mushroom teas, kinesiology: these are just a few of the many alternative therapies I've heard about from my patients, eager to protect themselves against cancer. While I can't fault these women for trying, many of the remedies sound too good to be true—especially to the cancer survivor who may have just finished the grueling ordeal of treatment.

At present, none of these unorthodox measures have ever been proven, at least in a true scientific way. Though some regimens appear to have potential, we still don't know enough about dosage levels or frequency of use, let alone any possible long-term side effects. Given all this uncertainty, it is still too soon to recommend any of these unorthodox remedies to stem the onset of cancer.

Future Preventions

In the near future, doctors hope to provide women with more specific remedies for preventing certain cancers. Evidence shows that aspirin may help stave off colon cancer by blocking the production of cyclooxygenase, an enzyme that fuels the growth of malignant tumors. Moreover, numerous studies have shown that folic acid, a B vitamin found in liver, beans, citrus fruits, and dark leafy vegetables, is linked to a decreased risk of breast cancer and precancerous colon polyps and may help lower the risk for cervical dysplasia.

The most encouraging research to date, however, comes from Italian studies that have found that certain natural and synthetic forms of vitamin A called retinoids may have a protective effect against breast cancer.

Despite these promising finds, more study is needed to determine the most effective dosage and schedule of these anticancer substances. But doctors expect that in the next few years, some or all of them will become part of a new arsenal of chemopreventatives in the fight to eliminate cancer.

Until then, the best way of limiting your risks is to eat a balanced and healthy diet, get plenty of exercise, and eliminate your bad health habits. Though there are no guarantees that switching to a healthier lifestyle will prevent cancer or any other major disease from occurring, it certainly can't hurt. More and more, studies show that people who exercise regularly and eat the proper foods, low in fat and high in fresh fruits and vegetables, have a lower incidence of cancer as well as heart disease, diabetes, and other chronic diseases. The evidence is also clear that cutting out the bad behaviors like smoking and unprotected sun exposure can cut your risk.

So the message I give all cancer survivors is simple: If making these changes in your life will give you an added edge over cancer, then why not try? In doing so, you'll undoubtedly feel better and have a healthier outlook on life. And living is what surviving cancer is all about.

Five

COPING WITH PHYSICAL SCARS

*E*nding treatment with a clean bill of health is the hope of every cancer survivor. Yet few women emerge from the experience without some physical change. Perhaps the greatest irony of cancer therapy is that the methods used to destroy the disease can also damage the patient, forcing many women to contend with a host of disabling side effects as they struggle to resume their lives.

Although most of the effects from surgery, radiation, and chemotherapy eventually subside, it may take months or years for some symptoms to fade, and others may surface unexpectedly long after therapy is complete. Living day-to-day with these physical complications, and coping with their emotional aftermath, can have a devastating effect on a woman's self-esteem and body image. Even when her hair has grown back and her strength revived, a survivor may still face more lingering reminders of her ordeal and the toll it took to survive.

Learning to manage and adjust to these physical scars can make the victory over cancer seem in many ways a bittersweet one. Yet I prefer to see such compromises as a testament to the extraordinary strength and resiliency each survivor carries within her. Ask any woman who's had cancer how she coped through the grueling weeks and months of her therapy, and her answer is simple: "I just did." When a survivor suffers side effects, the answer is the same. Though the support of family and friends undoubtedly helps, a survivor's remarkable capacity to rebound from hardship is what really gets her through the bumps and potholes of life.

Still, there are times when even the strongest of women feel sad and hopeless. Every survivor has days when her worries about the future, her finances, and her problems of dealing with everyday affairs leave her longing tearfully for life as it was before. This is all part of the normal mourning each woman must go through to get beyond her cancer. However, it can help to remember that no matter how distressing the changes and scars to your body, there will always be ways to cope. Try to remember: the real "you" hasn't changed at all. Though some of the problems you may experience will be impossible to correct, others can be eliminated (or at least eased) through surgery, medication, or changes in your lifestyle.

This chapter will give you information on some of the major side effects to expect after treatment and offer strategies for living with the range of disabilities you may face. While you already may have heard about some of them from your physician, you could encounter others as you get farther away from treatment. Keep in mind that any new symptom or difficulty should be reported immediately to your doctor. Not every ache or cramp is a sign of disease. But the only way to know for certain is to get promptly and properly checked.

Facing the Effects of Surgery

To save a woman's life and prevent the deadly spread of cancer, surgeons must often remove important organs or tissues, leaving behind disfiguring scars or disabilities. Though most patients understand the reasoning behind this action, it can be a shock to view their own bodies changed, let alone contemplate the use of appliances or prostheses (artificial devices) that now may be necessary in their lives. Each of us develops an image about our body. While we may not always be completely satisfied with that image, it still remains part of who we are and how we are viewed by others. And when cancer forces a piece of it to be cut away—whether it be a breast, a uterus, or a part of one's bowel—it can feel as if a close friend or relative has died. A patient of mine who had her breast removed described her feelings as a deep, almost primal sense of loss; another patient who lost her uterus likened her first few months after surgery to a period of mourning. "I felt bereft and depressed, as if the root of my womanhood and femininity had been suddenly stripped away."

It may take some time to work through these normal feelings of grief. Fortunately, with advances in plastic surgery and the use of cosmetic and functional prostheses, many survivors are made to feel whole again or, at the very least, helped to better cope with the physical and emotional consequences of a lost body part. Most insurance companies cover restorative or cosmetic surgery and various prosthetic devices as a necessary part of the rehabilitation process. Once the treatment process is complete, your doctor can help you learn more about the kinds of reconstruction available for your specific situation if you so desire.

Gynecologic Cancer and Reconstruction

Generally, when a woman has a hysterectomy for cancer, she must have her uterus, cervix, fallopian tubes, and ovaries removed. When such drastic steps are taken, it can take weeks for the scars to heal and months for a woman's normal energy to return. Though physically and emotionally traumatic at any age, the experience can have devastating consequences for a woman who still hasn't completed her family. Having lost the source of her fertility and her ability to menstruate, she may feel robbed of the choice of motherhood. She also may be faced with the early and disturbing symptoms of menopause—hot flashes or vaginal dryness—making her feel old before her time. A woman who has already gone through menopause may feel equally devastated because the uterus symbolizes a woman's uniqueness—her ability to reproduce. She may feel this defined her as a woman.

At the same time, a woman may fear the operation will leave a massive and empty hole in her abdomen. In truth, however, the uterus is only about three and a half inches long by two and a half inches wide and gets smaller as a woman grows older. When it is removed the intestines naturally fill the space, while the vagina stays anchored to supporting ligaments that hold it in place.

Nevertheless, some women worry that after a hysterectomy they will lose the essence of their womanhood, get fat and hairy, or even develop a male voice as a consequence. But this is just a myth. As I try to explain to my patients—and their partners when appropriate—removing the uterus does not change a woman's character or her femininity. Nor does it interfere with her libido, with the enjoyment of intercourse, or with a woman's ability to reach orgasm. Despite the anatomical changes that occur from hysterectomy, the sensitivity of the clitoris does not diminish. Although a woman may have difficulty with vaginal lubrication, she can use over-the-counter products like Astroglide, Replens, or K-Y jelly to supplement her own secretions, or she may be placed on hormonal therapy. Providing she feels up to it, and her physician agrees, she'll be able to resume sexual relations as soon as six weeks after surgery. If the ovaries are not removed at the time of hysterectomy, a woman will not experience any hormonal changes. She will stop having periods, of course, but she will not have hot flashes or flushes.

On the other hand, some invasive cancers of the reproductive tract may require further surgery to remove the bladder, vagina, even the vulva. Fortunately, new procedures in plastic and reconstructive surgery can now restore these organs, enabling women to continue to function sexually. For example, if a woman's vagina needs to be removed because of cancer, a new vagina can be created from nearby muscle and skin. This "neovagina" will allow the woman to have intercourse, and since her clitoris remains intact, she can still have an orgasm (further discussed in chapter 6). Other techniques in plastic surgery can also eliminate the need for outside appliances: in a new procedure called continent urinary diversion, doctors can reconstruct a bladder out of a portion of a patient's bowel. Once completed, the woman is left only with a small pink "nipple" on the outside of her abdomen over which she can put a Band-Aid, removing it every few hours to catheterize herself and empty her new internal bladder.

Living with Ostomy Surgery

When cancer requires the removal of all or part of the colon (large intestines), a new opening may have to be created to permit the elimination of digestive waste. In this procedure a part of the bowel is passed through an incision in the abdomen and formed into a surgically created port called an ostomy, or stoma. Body wastes are then eliminated directly through the stoma into a special pouch called an appliance. Some survivors live permanently with their colostomies, while others are able eventually to have their stoma closed and their bowel reconnected. Each case is different, and you'll need to discuss with your doctor whether or not you can later have your colostomy closed.

But don't be discouraged if you can't. Though an inconvenient reminder of your cancer ordeal, a colostomy shouldn't impede you from being just as active and outgoing as you were before surgery. Thousands of survivors continue to work, engage in a variety of sports (including swimming!), and have fulfilling sexual relationships in spite of their colostomy.

Five years ago a patient of mine named Jackie developed familial colon cancer at the age of thirty-four, requiring the complete removal of her large bowel. Determined not to let cancer or its treatment get the better of her, Jackie has since married and had two beautiful children. At our last follow-up visit, she asked if I'd mind forwarding her a case of disposable pouches to Nepal. She was off for a three-month trek through the Himalayas and didn't have room in her suitcase for all her supplies.

"Are you having any problems with your appliance?" I asked.

"Oh, I hated it at first," she admitted. "Always worrying about it leaking or its smell. But once I got comfortable with a routine, and felt more confident, it became more of an inconvenience than an impediment. When people hear I have one, they always imagine it to be this great tragedy. But most of the time I forget it exists, and go about my life like anyone else."

As with anything new, living with a colostomy takes some getting used to. The look, size, shape, and location of the stoma vary from person to person, but in general stomas are strong and resilient. They cannot be injured during normal everyday events, such as showering or bumping into something. Before leaving the hospital, you probably received a thorough training on the two types of colostomy appliances available—the more expensive disposable pouches, which are discarded after several days, and reusable pouches, which can be cleaned and used repeatedly, provided good hygiene is observed.

At first, learning how to use this equipment may seem overwhelming and a bit depressing. While it's natural to worry about odor and leakage, such problems are much less likely to occur today than they were in the past. Today's appliances are made of sturdy materials and fit very securely; they can be deodorized with drops or powders. All survivors will suffer a mishap or two before they become adept at securing their appliance. But try to be patient. As time goes by, you'll learn how to avoid those embarrassing moments, perhaps even joke about them. If the colostomy is done on the lower part of your colon, you may be able to "train" your bowel to evacuate at certain times, which enables you to abandon wearing a bag. Your surgeon can advise you on where exactly your stoma was placed and if such retraining is possible.

Women who have had a colostomy do not require a special diet, although they may be advised to increase their fiber intake as an aid to both digestion and elimination. To prevent problems with intestinal gas, the intake of high-fiber foods should be increased gradually and foods that tend to produce a lot of flatulence should be avoided. Your physician can help you figure out which foods to include or avoid in your diet and whom to consult for proper care and selection of equipment.

Women with colostomies are usually able to remain just as sexually active as they were before their surgery. Speak with your physician about any problems or concerns you're having about sex. She may suggest you attend a support group where people with colostomies have a chance to compare notes and hear how others in the same situation deal with problems. For more information on living with a colostomy, contact the United Ostomy Association (see "Resources").

To smooth the way for "rookie" colostomy owners, my patients suggest having these essential items on hand:

- plenty of your favorite room freshener.
- small plastic garbage can and liners to discard materials that cannot be flushed down the toilet.
- a plastic container for soaking or bleaching your drainable pouches in some cleansing solution. Some of my patients use a little Lysol and bleach mixed with two quarts of water. But first consult your physician for advice.
- several rolls of paper towels for "stuffing" the drainable pouches after they've been rinsed. Be sure to use cold water, or they may take on the consistency of bubble gum.
- a plastic one-quart pitcher with handle to hold water to rinse out your pouch before you soak it in cleansing solution.
- baby oil for squirting into a fresh drainable pouch after the clamp is on, but *before* putting it onto your barrier. It allows fecal material to slide down the pouch rather than accumulate near the stoma.
- cotton-tipped swabs to gently clean away fecal material from around the stoma or from any "pockets" that may have formed in the barrier seal.
- a tube of dermal wound gel to apply to the stoma area every time you change the drainable pouch.
- a tube of barrier cream to completely clean your skin when the barrier is removed.
- a box of skin prep wipes in individual packages for use before the adhesive barrier is used.
- cuticle scissors for trimming the hole in the barrier to your exact size. Some already come with precut holes.
- an extra supply of pouch deodorants, barriers with flanges, and drainable pouches, plus a few extra plastic clamps for the drainable pouch.

Mastectomy and Reconstruction

No matter how much a woman reads about breast surgery or how much support she receives from relatives and friends, it never is enough to prepare her for the shock of looking down at her own mastectomy scar. Each survivor experiences a different and unique level of grief when she loses a breast to cancer. And every woman needs time to mourn her loss and reconcile her feelings. As an oncologist, and a breast cancer survivor myself, I know how important it is for family members, as well as doctors, to acknowledge this and respect it. As one survivor once put it:

> Losing a breast was like losing a photograph album of my children when they were young. The breast was a connection to their infancy and childhood, the source of their earliest nourishment, the pillow upon which they slept, and a haven when they were hurt or scared. It was also a haven for my husband—a place to rest his head when a day became too long or a night too sleepless. It was a symbol of shared intimacy, as well as a source of pleasure. And when that loss was recognized, I somehow felt validated.

We live in a society that worships breasts, not for their function, but for their form. Although some women choose to live proudly with the scars of mastectomy, others prefer to use a foam-filled prosthesis they can wear in their bra or pin to an undergarment. Still others feel it important to reconstruct the shape and look of a new breast. It is a personal decision that rests solely with the woman. And no decision should be considered too vain.

"Even though my husband told me he married *all* of me, not just my breasts, it was hard for me to believe him," says Peggy, a fifty-nine-year-old breast cancer survivor from Philadelphia. "To me the scar was a mutilation, and I couldn't look in the mirror without crying. I used to undress in the closet so he wouldn't see me. It was important for me to feel whole again, and now that my breast has been reconstructed, I do."

The decision to undergo reconstruction after mastectomy has to do with a woman's sense of self, with restoring what has been lost. It is not merely a question of vanity, but rather a need to put back what cancer took away. A husband may say, "It's you I love, not your breast"; a surgeon may poo-poo your concerns or chide you about feeling lucky to be alive. But if you're not happy living with your mastectomy, you are entitled to seek consultation and not have your feelings minimized because you want your breast restored.

Eventually, more than half the women treated with mastectomy decide to have their breasts reconstructed. While some elect to have the surgery at the same time as their mastectomy, others are advised by their doctors to wait until their treatment with chemotherapy is complete. A number of methods are possible: insertion of a saline- or fat-filled implant under the skin, or a procedure known as a myocutaneous flap, where tissue is transferred from the abdomen, back, or upper buttock, either to make a foundation for an implant or to serve as the breast itself. A small sliver of labial tissue is then fashioned into a nipple and a circular patch of dark skin from the inner thigh taken to form an areola. Such reconstructive surgery is expensive, but, unlike cosmetic operations, it is usually covered in part or completely by major medical insurance.

Until recently, silicone-filled implants were also used in many breast reconstructions. But when a number of complaints arose linking them to rheumatoid arthritis and other serious diseases, the Food and Drug Administration removed them from the market (except for use in very restricted settings). This action was widely interpreted as a judgment that the implants were dangerous, alarming many women who had already received them.

Numerous studies have since revealed that women who get silicone implants are no more likely than anyone else to develop arthritis, lupus, scleroderma, and other autoimmune diseases. Although this comes as encouraging news for women who already have these implants, it still doesn't mean that silicone implants pose no risk at all. While most experts feel the study was perhaps the best epidemiological research to date, critics still complain that they do not address other medical concerns associated with the implants, such as scarring, hardening and rupture of the implants, and inflammation and pain at the site of the implant, or fears that implants might interfere with mammography designed to detect breast cancer.

More research into these problem areas continues to be done. In the meantime, if you already have a silicone implant, you should discuss whether to remove it or leave it in place with your doctor.

On the other hand, if you have just begun to contemplate breast reconstruction, you'll need to have a consultation with your oncologist and several plastic surgeons. This way you can learn more about the various options available and the ideal course of treatment for you as an individual. Because each plastic surgeon has his own artistic preferences and styles, you should ask to see pictures of the breasts he's reconstructed. Usually he'll have a portfolio of photographs for you to look through and may even advise you to speak with some of his patients. Later, if you are happy with the results, he may ask to take a picture of you (from the neck down, of course), which can help other women in their decision-making process.

Before you proceed with reconstruction, however, you should know that the procedure cannot restore the sensitivity of your breast. Most cancer surgery damages sensitive nerves in that area that cannot be repaired. Even so, the skin over the breast will feel natural to the touch, and if abdominal tissue is used, the texture will be more like that of a normal breast.

After reconstruction you should continue to have regular follow-up exams with your oncologist and examine *both* of your breasts monthly. So far, there is no evidence that silicone or saline implants increase the risk of breast cancer. However, silicone implants may impede cancer detection by obscuring developing tumors on mammography. Radiologists are investigating the use of MRI (magnetic resonance imaging) and ultrasound to evaluate women who have these implants. It is important that your doctor examine the scar area of your mastectomy to look for signs of local recurrences. Generally, with regular physical exams and mammography, physicians will be able to spot return of disease, either beneath or around an implant.

Lumpectomy with Radiation

Lumpectomy, node dissection, and radiation is generally a far less mutilating alternative to mastectomy. Yet some lumpectomies may later require plastic surgery, especially when surgeons are forced to remove more cancerous tissue than originally intended. Once a woman's breast tissue has been irradiated, the blood supply to the area may be damaged or scarred, making it extremely difficult for a plastic surgeon to correct surgical deformities. In fact, when a lumpectomy has gone awry, most plastic surgeons find it easier to remove the breast and reconstruct a new one, rather than try to repair irradiated breast tissue.

When you developed breast cancer, your oncologist most likely discussed your alternatives for treatment and the kind of defect you'd be left with. But it's important to remain up-to-date on the success of various breast cancer therapies since there is always the chance of developing a second cancer in your breast or a recurrence in the breast that still remains.

Problems After Chemotherapy

Some cancers can be removed by surgery without the need for further treatment. But frequently chemotherapy must be employed in order to ensure that microscopic traces of the disease are destroyed. Unfortunately, most of the drugs used to kill malignant cells also end up destroying healthy and normal cells in the process. This can lead to a host of unpleasant side effects, many of which disappear after therapy is complete. On occasion, however, chemotherapy leaves more permanent scars, some of which occur only months or years later.

Numbness in the Hands and Feet

Neuropathy (nerve damage) can be one of the most disturbing consequences of chemotherapy. When Carol was fifty-two, she received cisplatin as part of an aggressive chemotherapy regimen for ovarian cancer. Five years later she remains cancer-free, but she still suffers from numbness in her hands and feet.

"Initially after treatment, I was frightened to walk," says the retired schoolteacher. "I was afraid of falling, especially when I went up or down steps. At first I needed help with everything—buttoning my coat, tying my shoes, getting out money for the bus. It was demoralizing, but with time the neuropathy has gotten better, and now I feel a lot more independent."

Chemotherapy-related neuropathies are commonly related to agents like cisplatin, vincristine, DTIC, and taxol. The nerve damage may not be evident until months after completion of treatment. It is impossible to predict how long a neuropathy will last or if it will go away at all. Generally, however, it will get better with time.

In learning to live with this problem, survivors need to take special care to avoid potential injuries from burns and sharp objects. They also should inspect their hands and feet daily for signs of infection that may have gone unnoticed. There are many products on the market to help with day-to-day tasks. Check the "Resources" section in the back of this book or ask your doctor for help. Physical therapy is often useful for strengthening the muscles in your arms and legs. Though neuropathies can be a major annoyance to live with and can even be quite debilitating, they don't have to impede you from enjoying a full and productive life.

Constipation

After chemotherapy, patients frequently complain about difficulty in moving their bowels. Certain drugs like vincristine and vinblastine can slow down and temporarily immobilize the peristaltic action of the bowel, which moves waste through the intestines. Narcotics, antidepressants, and other medications may also cause a slowing down of bowel function. In addition, constipation may be caused from dehydration or lack of adequate fiber in the diet. Many women experience some sort of irregularity soon after treatment, but this often resolves itself once they increase the fiber in their diet and begin drinking at least eight to ten glasses of water a day.

However, some of my patients find constipation to be a more chronic problem. Often they have to relearn how to have a bowel movement, making sure they respond immediately to the urge to defecate, preferably in a private environment that reduces distraction. If they still have problems, I recommend taking one or two Senokot (senna concentrate) tablets daily as a natural laxative. If this doesn't help, they may need a stronger medication temporarily. However, prolonged use of laxatives or enemas can inhibit the body's natural ability to have a bowel movement. Check with your physician if constipation persists or you experience sudden or severe abdominal cramps. These could be signs of appendicitis, diverticulitis, gallstones, or a recurrence of pelvic disease, which require immediate treatment.

Heart, Lung, and Kidney Damage

Some anticancer drugs may cause long-term problems to otherwise healthy organs. Cisplatin can produce kidney damage and hearing problems, including tinnitus (ringing in the ears) and hearing loss. Commonly used antitumor antibiotics like Adriamycin may cause heart damage that in turn may lead to chronic congestive heart failure. Bleomycin may cause lung damage.

Not every woman who's been treated with these medications develops later complications. If your health was good before treatment, you are probably at minimal risk. However, older women with a history of hypertension, coronary heart disease, or lung disease may need to be monitored more closely.

If you've taken cardiotoxic medications, be sure your physician performs a periodic electrocardiogram (EKG) and one follow-up "ejection fraction" test to determine the muscle damage to your heart, if any. Cumulative heart failure can take years to develop and may be triggered by periods of extreme stress, such as pregnancy or vigorous exercise. Notify your physician if you develop symptoms like shortness of breath, swelling of the legs or feet, inability to tolerate exercise, a fast and irregular heartbeat, wheezing, and, in some cases, chest pain. If problems occur, you may be placed on a heart medication like digitalis to minimize your symptoms and prevent further damage. A seventy-two-year-old patient of mine had been treated ten years earlier with Adriamycin for ovarian cancer. Although she was cured of her cancer, she later developed coronary artery disease. Since the Adriamycin had caused heart muscle damage, the decreased blood flow from coronary heart disease resulted in her developing shortness of breath and a rapid heart rate from congestive heart failure. She was treated with diuretics, digoxin, and other cardiac medications, and fortunately her symptoms improved.

In another instance recently, a twenty-six-year-old patient named Crystal came in for a regular follow-up, complaining that she just didn't feel herself. "I know it sounds silly, but I can't stop yawning at work," she explained. "I feel tired all the time, and when I climb the flight of stairs to my apartment, I have to stop and catch my breath."

On examination, I discovered that Crystal was suffering the beginning stages of pulmonary fibrosis, a scarring of the lungs that sometimes results from treatment with bleomycin, which she'd received as a teenager for a germ cell tumor of her ovary. Fortunately, with medication her breathing became easier. But she would need to guard against respiratory infections and take care not to exercise too vigorously. "How strange that after all this time, cancer is still running my life," she told me, a bit discouraged. "But I guess I have to feel lucky that I've been given a second chance to stay healthy."

Damage from Radiation

Generally, most of the acute side effects of radiation treatment are confined to the part of the body that was irradiated. While problems like skin burns, fatigue, and upset bowels are usually short-lived, others may be longer lasting or surface months or years after recovery.

Perception and Memory Loss

After twenty-six-year-old Tricia began suffering severe headaches and blurred vision two years ago, she was diagnosed with gestational trophoblastic disease, a cancer of the placenta that had spread to her brain. She underwent cranial radiation and chemotherapy. But several months into her recovery, Tricia began to notice strange effects from her treatment.

"A couple of times I forgot to meet friends for lunch," she recalls. "Then one evening, I was walking home from my mother's house, and the next thing I knew, I was standing in the middle of my kitchen. I couldn't remember how I got there, and I started to get scared."

Many women who receive radiation to the brain or central nervous system experience some degree of memory loss or perception and occasionally may suffer a drop in their IQ level or diminished motor skills. Although some effects can be permanent, others may be more remedial in nature and correctable with occupational and physical rehabilitation. Often it depends on the dosage of the radiation and the location of the treatment. Your doctor is the best person to evaluate the extent of the damage and how it can be managed most effectively.

Pain and Scarring

Some survivors develop chronic pain as a consequence of treatment. This usually occurs in a part of the body where surgery and radiation have been used together, leading to the development of scar tissue, which entraps and injures the adjacent nerves. After lumpectomy with radiation, a survivor may occasionally suffer a referred pain down her arm, especially in warm, humid weather. This is usually relieved by massaging the arm gently and taking nonprescription painkillers like acetaminophen (Tylenol) or ibuprofen. More severe cases of radiation scarring may require the use of exercise, splinting, orthotic appliances, or surgery to cut away the scarring.

Radiation to the neck and chest can also cause scarring of the thyroid gland, a crucial organ that regulates body metabolism. Hypothyroidism (low thyroid function) occurs in up to a quarter of all patients given full-dose mantle irradiation, and its major symptoms include lethargy, inability to concentrate, depression, weight gain, dry and scaly skin, and a loss of hair, particularly along the eyebrows. Radiation may also cause the reverse condition, known as hyperthyroidism, which leads to heart palpitations, sudden loss of weight, nervousness, muscle weakness, even eye problems. Both conditions are easily treated if diagnosed early.

If you've undergone radiation to your neck, be sure you have your thyroid gland checked at each follow-up examination. A simple blood test can easily diagnose problems and should be repeated at least once a year.

Dry Mouth

Xerostomia (dry mouth) is a common and sometimes permanent consequence of having radiation to the neck or chest area. Even if the problem is temporary, a woman's production of saliva may not reach its usual level for six months to a year after treatment. As a result, you may have irritated gums and teeth, a diminished sense of taste (since food must be in a solution to be tasted), difficulty chewing, and trouble enunciating your words.

To relieve your symptoms, drink water or nonirritating fruit juices several times an hour. In between, moisten your lips with Vaseline or lip balm and suck on smooth, flat candies or lozenges to stimulate saliva production. An over-the-counter remedy called Papain is sometimes helpful for dissolving thick oral secretions and can be swabbed in the mouth before eating. If your symptoms become severe or you cease to produce any saliva, your physician may prescribe a medication called pilocarpine, which often brings relief by stimulating the flow of saliva.

Because xerostomia interferes with taste, you also may need to modify your diet to make foods more flavorful but less spicy. With persistent mouth dryness and irritation, it's best to stick with moist, soft, or smooth foods such as buttered noodles, puddings, yogurt, ices, hot or cold soups, juice, or purees.

Survivors who have undergone radiation to the head or neck also need to be especially careful with their dental care. Regular brushing and flossing, combined with prophylactic treatments with fluoride from the dentist, are the best ways to prevent tooth damage and infection.

Diarrhea

Chronic diarrhea is an embarrassing and sometimes dangerous side effect of pelvic radiation. If left untreated, it can cause dizziness and dehydration, eventually leading to kidney damage and severe metabolic problems. Often, over-the-counter medications like Kaopectate, Pepto-Bismol, or Imodium can alleviate mild symptoms. But if you find you are having frequent loose stools for over a week, contact your physician. She may recommend a medication like Lomotil or paragoric to slow down your bowels and ask you to increase your fluids, especially fruit juices and Gatorade, which will help restore sodium, potassium, and other important minerals that may be lost. She will also check your stool for infection. *Clostridium dificile* is bacteria that commonly causes diarrhea in patients who have received radiation or chemotherapy. However, because this infection can be lethal if unattended, you should notify your doctor immediately about any problems with diarrhea. She can prescribe antibiotics that will easily kill the infection and alleviate its symptoms.

Problems with diarrhea may be helped by a diet that is high in calories and protein but low in fat and fiber. Instead of three large meals a day, try eating smaller portions more frequently. Eat foods that are warm or at room temperature. After each bowel movement, cleanse the area with warm water and a mild soap like Dove or Ivory liquid, then rinse and pat dry. A local anesthetic in spray or ointment can relieve a persistent itch or tenderness in the anal region; Sween Cream, a nonprescription ointment, may also prevent irritation. But you may want to wear a sanitary napkin or product like Assure to avoid the embarrassment of incontinence.

Several of my patients who have had pelvic radiation complain of chronic diarrhea and occasional bloody stools. I usually refer them to a gastroenterologist to make sure their complaints are related to the radiation treatments and not a new problem, like polyps, hemorrhoids, or even a second cancer. Often the gastroenterologist will prescribe a regimen of diet and medication that will control the symptoms.

Lymphedema

When lymph nodes are removed or damaged because of surgery or radiation, a chronic swelling in the arm or in the leg can result. This is called lymphedema and most often occurs in women who have had breast or vulvar surgery with lymph node dissection and radiation. The condition may be painless or painful. It also can be disfiguring and may have serious consequences if a cut or abrasion on the affected limb causes a subsequent infection. The lymph nodes act as "filters" to prevent infection. Without them your body is less able to fight off bacteria and disease, particularly in the affected limb.

Last summer Judy, a fifty-three-year-old magazine editor, came to see me for a lesion on her vulva. A biopsy of her left labia revealed vulvar cancer, and I immediately performed a radical wide local excision of her vulva and removal of her left groin lymph nodes. Three of the lymph nodes tested positive, so I recommended a course of pelvic radiation treatments. Judy was relieved to know her cancer was under control and within several months was able to return to work. But one afternoon she called me, crying and upset.

"I can barely walk," she said. "My left leg is swollen and puffy, and my shoes won't fit." When she came to my office the following day, I explained she had lymphedema and that the swelling was due to a buildup of lymphatic fluid. I suggested she try to control it with a tight compression stocking and that she be careful not to injure her legs or feet in any way. Even an insect bite or hangnail could lead to serious infection.

The next day she visited a physical therapist who showed her how to use a special compression pump that controlled the lymphedema by keeping lymphatic fluid circulating. Now she uses the pump two times a week and wears heavy support stockings during the day. Though neither have been able to cure Judy's condition entirely, they have made it more tolerable and a good deal safer in the long run.

To avoid problems following a lymph node dissection (for example, with breast cancer or vulvar cancer), always take special care to protect yourself from sunburns, use insect repellent outdoors, and wear gloves for housework and gardening. Use an electric razor with a narrow head for shaving to reduce the risk of nicks and scratches. And *never* cut your cuticles. If you do get a cut or abrasion on the affected limb, wash the area immediately with soap and water, apply an antibacterial medication, and cover it with a bandage, watching carefully for redness, soreness, or other signs of infection. In addition, be sure that any injections, vaccinations, blood samples, or blood pressure tests are done on your unaffected limb whenever possible. You also may want to invest in a medical tag identifying your condition in the event of an accident or emergency.

If you develop lymphedema, it's also advisable not to wear any confining jewelry or cuffs around the affected limb, and try to rest the area in an elevated position whenever possible to relieve swelling. Compression garments should always be worn over the entire extent of the swelling. A stocking that reaches only to the knee tends to develop tightness and can exacerbate any swelling that develops in the thigh. Ready-made garments are available in a variety of sizes (see "Resources") and should not be confused with the thin support hose that are generally ineffective in the management of swelling. If your lymphedema is long-standing, you may want to consider a custom-made compressive garment. The one major drawback of these elastic garments is that they are extremely difficult to get on and off. A newer, nonelastic compressive orthotic, which consists of a series of adjustable straps, is much easier to apply, but it looks pretty unsightly.

Unfortunately, in some women a compressive garment alone is not sufficient to manage severe lymphedema. For these survivors, a compression pump of the kind Judy used often helps. It consists of an inflatable tube that goes around the limb and cyclically fills with air, pressing fluid out of the affected area. Some women find it most successful to use the pump at home on a nightly basis and wear a compressive sleeve or stocking during the day. But before you consider the pump, consult your physician.

Most important, if you suddenly notice a problem with swelling, or your arm or legs become red or hot, call your doctor. Most problems are treatable, but there may be underlying causes of infection or clots in veins that warrant prompt and thorough investigation by your oncologist.

Chronic Fatigue

After treatment it's common to feel exhausted and spent. No one comes through an ordeal as traumatic as cancer and jumps right back into life. Every survivor experiences feelings of uncertainty and depression about the days that lie ahead. Patients have to reconcile feelings of confronting their own mortality, and they have to learn to accommodate to the long-term physical effects of their treatment. As a result, it's only normal to feel tired and a bit run-down. But there also may be physiological reasons why some women feel so weary and worn out.

Although experts still haven't pinned down an exact cause for chronic fatigue, some believe it is brought about by the additional energy the body must expend on repairing injured cells. Others suspect that bone marrow suppression is responsible. When your body produces fewer white cells to fight infection, fewer red cells to carry oxygen (anemia), and fewer platelets to assist blood clotting, you can end up exhausted.

Every survivor needs time to recover after treatment; at first you may have to make some compromises in your routine or learn to accept a different level of activity. If your friends and family want to pamper you, let them. They may not cook every meal the way you like, or clean the house just right, but their help will give you time to relax and allow your body to heal. If you feel guilty about not getting back to the office, try to arrange a flexible schedule that lets you work several days at home. If your kids are tiring you out, take them to the movies or drop them at a friend's house.

It's important to take time for yourself and give yourself permission to rest. In the beginning you may want to nap once or twice a day so you can enjoy time with your family at night. If napping doesn't suit you, try other forms of relaxation like reading, listening to music, or a gentle stretching routine. Exercise is an excellent way to build up strength and stamina after treatment and often can be a wonderful outlet for the emotions as well. However, you should wait four to six weeks after therapy before starting a program, and always check first with your doctor. "I may not always look great doing it, but it sure feels good," says one of my breast cancer patients who took up ballet after her mastectomy. "Now I do everything possible to make the present happy, and if that means taking time for myself, so be it."

Living with Compromise

To the outside world, surviving cancer implies being cured, winning the battle over life-threatening disease, and returning to a healthy and active life. Yet frequently many women are discouraged to find that after treatment they actually feel worse than when they started, at least for a while. Coming to terms with the physical realities of treatment can take a long time, sometimes years. Accepting who you've become while learning to live with disability or disfigurement is a difficult, sometimes overwhelming challenge. Can I accept the body I've been left with? Will I ever return to normal? Will my partner still need me, love me, want me, now that my image has changed? Sorting through these issues can be the hardest part of coping—one that many survivors approach with a great deal of bitterness and rage.

Several years ago I treated a forty-year-old Jordanian immigrant named Petra for advanced ovarian cancer. After a full hysterectomy and surgical removal of her ovaries, she received six months of chemotherapy with cisplatin, eventually developing such severe nerve damage in her hands that she was forced to quit work as a seamstress. Uninsured and jobless, Petra borrowed money to continue treatment, seeing it as her only way to stay alive. But after two more cycles, her blood counts fell dangerously low. Before going on with chemotherapy, I needed to see if her cancer still existed, so I scheduled her for a second-look surgery. Only one lymph node proved positive for cancer. She'd had a major response to therapy. But when I told her that she still had persistent disease and would need more treatment, she was furious. "This really stinks," she said bitterly. "I'm broke, and I can't feel my hands. And still you tell me there's cancer!"

Petra had been willing to go through anything—lose her hair, her job, the feeling in her hands—to rid herself of cancer. But when she learned she still had the disease, it all seemed a terrible waste. Today Petra is off chemotherapy and in remission. But like many survivors, she'd felt a sense of anger and bitterness about the side effects of treatment. They resent the toll it can take on their spirit as well as their health. But when they consider the alternative, they realize there really is no other choice.

Do you give a woman toxic chemicals to cure her cancer, knowing they can cause nerve damage and swelling so she'll never hold her grandchild? Or do you treat her with less effective drugs, eventually watching her die before the infant is ever born? This is the terrible trade-off that patients and their doctors have to face, with survival the only option. However, the encouraging news is that newer drugs have fewer side effects, and doctors now have medications for preventing many of the ill effects of treatment. Scientists also are developing miniature antibodies small enough to elude the body's immune system and latch on to the surface of mutated genes, blocking them from activating the cancer process. These antibodies still are not ready for clinical testing, but other specialists are working on ways to target anticancer drugs directly to the tumor site, virtually eliminating the debilitating side effects on healthy, normal cells. In the next few years doctors hope to offer blood tests that will determine whether cancer is about to spread—and whether additional chemotherapy is really warranted. I predict that within the next two decades chemotherapy will become obsolete as doctors learn to short-circuit the specific genes responsible for cancer.

What good is this for women who have already battled cancer and survived? Plenty. Every person is at risk for cancer, particularly those who have suffered it in the past. No doubt you are concerned about the genetic component of your disease and the dangerous legacy you may be leaving to your daughters and future generations. In the next few years gene therapy is sure to become a part of the armamentarium against cancer. And as such, you may be able to benefit because of the potential for your developing second cancers or recurrence in your lifetime. If not, your children certainly will.

Your oncologist can keep you up-to-date with all these new developments and make sure you are screened properly for future disease. If you move away and need to see another physician, she can go over any current or future concerns about your health by phone and refer you to a physician in your new location. But in the end, it will be your strength and your courage to survive that empowers you to make it through life in spite of the scars that remain. For though you may not look or function exactly the way you used to, you can still learn to cope and continue on, working, playing, stumbling, dreaming, a bit differently from other women, perhaps, but nonetheless *alive*.

Six

SEX AFTER CANCER

For twenty-two years of marriage, Clara and Herb had always had a great sex life. They enjoyed giving each other pleasure and made a point of exploring new and exciting ways to rekindle their marital passion. Though their lives were sometimes hectic from juggling the responsibilities of three teenage children and two full-time jobs, they still made time to close their bedroom door, eager to relax in the intimacy that a long relationship can bring.

"Our friends used to call us the love birds," says Clara. "We were always holding hands, or smiling in a certain way at each other. But now . . ."

Clara's voice trails off as she looks down at her chest. Two years ago a routine mammogram revealed a small but aggressive tumor in her right breast. After a mastectomy and six months of chemotherapy, Clara came home cancer-free.

"But somehow the desire for closeness and sex was gone," she says. "I just didn't feel like a woman anymore."

After cancer many woman begin to doubt their sexuality and their appeal. Suddenly they find themselves wondering if they are still "whole" women. Physical realities—the loss of a breast, scars left by surgery, radiation damage—often give way to enormous questions of sexual self-worth and the importance our culture places upon physical appearance and body image. A survivor wants to return to a healthy and active sex life, and to accept her body postcancer, but she might suddenly begin wondering, "Does my partner still want me without my breast? Do I think I'm sexy?"

Sometimes the invisibility of a woman's physical scars can make survivorship even more difficult. This is especially true for women who have survived ovarian, uterine, and cervical cancer. The geography of these cancers leaves many women grappling with a disturbing sense of mystery—a glance in the mirror does not show the survivor, or her partner, the extent of damage her body has suffered. This unrest can move survivors to ask one of the most agonizing questions of all: "Do I still function sexually?"

Instead of speaking openly about these fears and concerns, many couples hide behind a wall of silence. Often husbands will hesitate to initiate sex, afraid that contact may further hurt or damage the woman in some way. The wife, who may already be wondering how desirable she is, will take this hesitation as justification that she is somehow damaged or unappealing. By not discussing their feelings, a woman and her partner may find themselves embroiled in a vicious cycle of misunderstanding, potentially placing their marriage or relationship in serious jeopardy.

And what of the cancer survivor who is single and without a committed sexual partner? How does she tell a potential lover that she has had cancer? And when does she reveal that the disease and its treatment has left her with only one breast, an ostomy bag, or unable to have children?

No matter how open-minded or liberated our society has become, sex after cancer still remains a difficult and often hidden issue. Few survivors ever ask about it, many couples simply stop having it, and often doctors are so awkward discussing it that they neglect to give their patients any useful information at all about how to enjoy an intimate relationship with their partner after their disease. In fact, so little information is available to survivors about sex after cancer that it ends up reinforcing the age-old myth that once a woman has had cancer, her ability to have sex and enjoy it is next to impossible.

But let's set the record straight. Sex *can* and *does* continue after cancer. A woman's need and desire for sex and intimacy does not diminish once she has gone through treatment. Although some couples may encounter initial problems having intercourse, these are not insurmountable. As long as a woman and her partner are willing to discuss their feelings and make some minor adjustments in the ways they engage in sex, lovemaking can still be as sensual and satisfying as it was before cancer. In fact, when a woman and her lover have faced the ordeal of cancer together, their newfound appreciation for life sometimes brings them closer than ever before.

Of course, there will be times when neither you nor your partner will feel like being intimate. But there are many ways to preserve a caring and affectionate relationship without having intercourse. The key is asking for what you want and keeping the channels of communication open. To help you get started, let's discuss some of the specific concerns many survivors have relating to sexuality and cancer, taking into account, of course, that sex between two people is *not* something to be performed out of duty or obligation, but rather is an act of love and tenderness to be shared and enjoyed.

Dispelling the Myths

Many myths surround the issue of cancer and sexuality, and before we go any farther we should look at the facts. For the record, cancer is not contagious or infectious. You cannot catch cancer from kissing, touching, or having sex with someone who has had the disease. Nor does resuming sex after treatment increase a woman's chances of a recurrence. Unlike AIDS or herpes, cancer is not sexually transmittable. A cancer cell from one person's body simply cannot take root and grow in someone else.

Two years ago, when I began telling patients that I had breast cancer, a husband told me, "See, I knew it was catching. Now my wife has gone and given you her disease." But he was wrong. There is no way to know for certain what specifically causes any cancer to develop. It may be a combination of what a woman eats, what genes she inherited, and which bad behaviors like smoking she still engages in, or it may be a simple case of bad luck. But getting cancer has absolutely nothing to do with catching it from someone else—or passing it along to your partner during sex.

On the other hand, after a woman has had cancer, she may stop having sex because she fears that the disease was caused by some sexual transgression in her past. Some women feel a sense of guilt and regret about having cancer of the ovary or uterus, believing it resulted from their being too "oversexed" or sexually promiscuous. Other women worry that their breast cancer was caused by too much fondling and caressing during sex. There are even survivors who see their cancer as a punishment for being raped, for having an extramarital affair, or for being sexually abused as a child. None of these associations are true.

Cancer is simply a random disease—albeit a devastating one—that can magnify any sexual troubles or insecurities that existed prior to diagnosis. Studies have shown that if a survivor had difficulties with sex before cancer, she may find them compounded after recovery. For example, take the case of Gina, a forty-eight-year-old survivor of ovarian cancer, who came to see me several months ago, complaining that she felt anxious and upset whenever her husband wanted sex. Though I suspected some of the problem stemmed from premature menopause and her inexperience with using artificial lubrication, I still thought she should see a psychiatrist on my staff for further counseling.

Eventually, after several sessions, Gina was able to reveal her deep-seated fear that being molested as a child was somehow connected to her getting cancer. "Just hearing my husband's footsteps on the way to the bedroom reminds me of the fear and dread I'd felt as a little girl," she told the therapist. Fortunately, with further counseling Gina and her husband were able to surmount these difficulties and eventually resume a satisfying sexual relationship. But as Gina explained to me at her last checkup: "Cancer has a strange way of shaking loose the monsters in your head. When your mind isn't ready for sex, there's no way your body will be, either."

Adjusting to Your New Body

Cancer is a trauma to any woman and her partner, and it may take weeks, if not months, for emotions to settle and a feeling of sexual desire to resurface. At first a survivor is too shell-shocked from treatment even to think about sex. She's exhausted and spent, unsure of her health and uncertain how her changed body will function. She's brushed up against her own mortality, and she needs to consolidate her feelings about the life she's left behind and the one that lies before her. There may be worries about finances, children to deal with, and a career to consider. Those first few weeks of recovery can seem like an overwhelming blur, a time when many survivors feel stunned and a bit numbed to the world that whirls around them.

But slowly, as the days pass and the crisis of cancer drifts farther away, other concerns begin to reemerge—perhaps none more basic than a woman's self-image. How she feels about herself as a woman, about her body and its ability to function normally, can play a major role in how quickly a survivor feels interested and willing to resume sexual activity. If a woman feels good about herself, despite her physical changes, her desire for sex may resurface as soon as her scars have healed. But if she worries that her partner will be turned off by her altered body, she may never feel excited or aroused.

Adjusting to a body change is sometimes the most difficult part of surviving cancer. In our society women are made to believe that their bodies, and in particular their genital organs, determine their female role. In turn, their value as women and as sexual partners is, to a great extent, determined by having these organs and how well they function. When a woman loses her breast to cancer, it threatens her femininity and her sexual attractiveness. If her uterus or ovaries are taken away, she may feel her sense of womanhood has been robbed as well. From a physical standpoint, none of these physical changes need to affect sexual function. But emotionally they can be traumatizing to deal with.

"All my life, whenever I'd meet a man, the first thing he'd focus in on was my chest," says Laura, a thirty-seven-year-old breast cancer survivor. "I was a forty-D and always getting compliments like, 'Gee, you have great boobs.' Not that I was wrapped up solely in my breasts. But they were part of my identity, part of what made me feel sexy and attractive. When cancer took one away, I was devastated."

Even temporary changes like the loss of your hair, a swollen arm, or fatigue can erode your good feelings about your physical appeal. If you see yourself as unattractive, you might anticipate rejection and avoid physical contact with your partner. In turn, he may take this as a sign that sexually you're no longer interested. "The first few nights I undressed in the bathroom," says Freddi, a forty-nine-year-old breast cancer survivor. "I made sure never to let my husband see me tending to the incision, or putting on the prosthesis. I wanted him to touch me, but I was afraid he'd be turned off by how I looked. But he must have sensed my insecurity because one night after dinner, he asked to see the scar."

Showing one's changed body to one's partner can be the moment of truth for many survivors, and women have to prepare themselves for how that's going to feel. Looking at a chest with only one breast or the scars from pelvic surgery can be startling at first. But these are caveats of cancer that a woman and her partner must learn to live with.

My husband, Sheldon, has never seemed to notice my scars, even though parts of my body look like a road map. There's the incision from my lumpectomy, the notches of subsequent biopsies, even a patch on my back the size of a golf ball from where a basal cell skin cancer was removed. But our relationship is grounded on more than skin-deep beauty. I know that my identity as a good doctor, a good wife, and a good lover comes not from whether I have scars or not; it comes from inside of me, from working hard, from being smart, from caring and loving and being a decent human being. My physical scars don't bother me or my husband because our lives have gone on in spite of my cancer.

But if you still have trouble feeling positive about your self-image, several approaches may be taken. Often, as already mentioned, women who have undergone mastectomy choose to have their breast reconstructed through plastic surgery. "It made me feel like more of a 'total' woman and allowed me to avoid many of the problems I could have had in the bedroom," says Judith, a forty-two-year-old book editor, who opted to have her breast restored six weeks after her chemotherapy ended. Other women prefer to use artificial breast forms and shop for the best prosthesis they can find; still others view their altered body as a badge of courage and forgo breast replacement altogether.

Each survivor needs to make a decision that feels right for her, even if it seems vain or narcissistic. But whatever step you take, you need to open the lines of communication with your partner and openly discuss your feelings and concerns. It may seem terrifying or a bit awkward at first, but you need to give him the signal that you're still interested in an intimate relationship. It's only normal to be apprehensive and unsure about yourself and your body after cancer. But eventually most couples come around to the stage of accommodation and adjustment and relearn how to share and enjoy their bodies again.

On occasion, though, there may be times your husband or partner seems to withdraw emotionally. Perhaps he feels uneasy or put off by the physical changes he sees. Perhaps he feels angry about how his life has changed or vulnerable about his own health concerns. In our culture men are not conditioned to discuss their emotions as readily as women. Be patient and give him some time to adjust and work out the issues on his own. If it's been a while, and he's still reacting negatively or unable to provide any physical reassurance that he loves you, it may be time to see a professional counselor. Couples who had problems in their sex life before cancer often find them compounded during recovery. And sometimes the only way to a better relationship is to ask for help.

Talk to Your Doctor

Talking to your doctor can help you get a sense of how your sex life may change after cancer. When you know what to expect, you can plan ways of dealing with those issues. But surprisingly few patients actually raise the issue of sexuality. As an oncologist, I find it striking that women are able to talk about how they are feeling, about their side effects from treatment, about their diets, their hair, their fears of recurrence, but rarely, if ever, do they ask for help in resolving particular sexual problems. If their partners join them for an office visit, they smile confidently and may ask a few questions, but certainly never about sex.

When it comes to discussing sex after cancer, most survivors keep the door to their bedroom closed. In general many feel too embarrassed or inhibited to talk about their own sexual needs and those of their partner. Some may have grown up in a repressive family where sex was never discussed. Others may have had unsatisfactory sexual relationships for their entire lives and see cancer as an excuse to end their sexual involvement. Still others, because of religious or social influences, believe that sexual activity is inappropriate except for the purpose of reproduction.

Consequently it is up to the physician to introduce the subject. But, unfortunately, few doctors actually do. Too often they just don't have the time to ask the one or two questions to get the conversation going. They also may feel awkward or hesitant to raise the issue of sex because they fear they will not have remedies to offer for a patient's specific problem. As a result, women too often find themselves in a gray zone of uncertainty, not knowing whether sex is possible, let alone their options for preserving and improving their sexuality.

Last year I removed a malignant tumor from the uterus of a seventy-eight-year-old woman named Sadie. A lovely, petite woman with a sparkling smile, Sadie had never spent a day away from her husband in fifty-five years of marriage—until cancer, that is. Fortunately her disease was slow growing, and after five days in the hospital I happily sent her home, disease-free. However, two months after her surgery, her husband called my office to say Sadie seemed very depressed and asked if I could talk with her. We met, and after fifteen minutes of sidestepping the issue, Sadie finally revealed that she and her husband were having sexual problems.

"He's afraid intercourse will hurt me, so now all he wants is oral sex," she said in a whisper.

This was very distasteful to Sadie, but she still consented, somehow thinking it was her duty to satisfy him. For the next half hour we talked about sex, probably the longest discussion Sadie had ever had about the issue. She told me what her sexual experience had been, and that while she sometimes had pleasure, she'd always felt a bit frustrated and unsatisfied at her end. So we discussed other ways she and her husband might enjoy intimacy beyond having oral sex, and within several weeks she called me back, a changed and happy woman.

Like many survivors, Sadie had somehow needed "permission" to express her sexual desires, and discussing her problems with a physician had made that possible. Women need to know that a physician is there not only to solve health problems, but also to provide appropriate counseling and treatment for sexual problems. If your doctor doesn't bring up the issue of sex, it's your obligation to do so. If you feel reluctant because your doctor is a man, try speaking with his nurse. Although she may not have the training to give specific advice, she can make a note in the chart to have your doctor talk to you more fully. If you don't understand something, ask your doctor to draw you a picture or use a model to explain how a part of your body may have changed because of the disease or its treatment. You need to know that losing a body part doesn't necessarily preclude a satisfying sexual experience. You may even want to ask your partner to visit the doctor with you to help allay his own anxieties and misconceptions.

Sometimes, however, oncologists aren't necessarily the right doctors to talk to about issues of sexuality. You may need to visit your gynecologist, who often has a broader training in caring for women's sexual concerns. These days women are often interested in knowing whether it's safe and appropriate to take hormone replacement therapy. This is a perfect way of opening up the topic of sexuality and raising such questions as "When can I start having intercourse again?" or "How can I avoid vaginal dryness?" These are questions all women ask themselves, and a survivor deserves to have her physician answer them in a thorough and candid fashion.

Invisible Wounds

Cancer of a woman's reproductive organs can have a tremendous impact on a woman's emotions. It can affect the most sensitive and personal aspects of her life, not only removing her capacity to have children, but leaving her with anatomical scars in her most sensitive sex organs. However, in recent years the emphasis in gynecologic oncology has been not only to limit the debilitating aspects of surgery, but also to emphasize the option of reconstructive techniques. For a woman whose past cancer surgery has left her sexually disabled, means are now available to repair the damage and give her back the ability to engage in a more fulfilling relationship.

Hysterectomy

A hysterectomy is most often employed to treat cancer of the uterus, ovaries, and fallopian tubes as well as cervical tumors. The surgeon removes the uterus and ligaments that hold it in place in the pelvis. Also removed is the cervix and an inch or two of the vagina around the cervix. Although the vagina is shortened, the area around the clitoris and the lining of the vagina remains as sensitive as before.

Many women who undergo a hysterectomy fear that they will lose their femininity along with their uterus. I try to explain to my patients, and their husbands when appropriate, that the uterus has nothing to do with sexual desire and nothing to do with the enjoyment of intercourse or the ability to reach orgasm. The only changes a woman will experience after having a hysterectomy are losing fertility and no longer menstruating. If a woman is in her thirties and forties and must have her ovaries removed—a procedure called salpingo-oophorectomy—she undoubtedly will experience symptoms of premature menopause, including vaginal dryness. She will need to use artificial lubricating products like Replens or Astroglide to replenish the moisture in her vagina before intercourse. But her sensations of pleasure will in no way be affected.

The idea that menopause always leads to depression and decreased sexual desire is a long-standing misconception. No scientific literature exists to support either of these widely held beliefs. Not only do many postmenopausal women enjoy active and fulfilling sex lives, but studies have shown they are less likely than premenopausal women to suffer from major depression.

Still, hysterectomy is a major surgical procedure that requires a four- to five-week recovery. During this time, intense physical exertion and sexual intercourse must be avoided. Your physician can tell you when it is safe to resume having sex and recommend different sexual positions to avoid discomfort or pain.

Pelvic Exenteration

Total pelvic exenteration is the most radical form of pelvic surgery. It most often is used when cancer of the cervix has recurred, despite prior surgery and radiation. The uterus, ovaries, cervix, vagina, bladder, urethra, and rectum are removed. At the same time, the bladder and vagina are usually reconstructed from skin grafts, while an ostomy may be created for the evacuation of stool.

It takes a long time to recover from pelvic exenteration, and many patients admit that they really don't feel themselves until a year after surgery. But given time, a woman can resume an active and pleasurable sex life, able to be aroused sexually and reach orgasm if her outer genitals, including the clitoris, are not removed.

When cancer surgery requires the removal of part or all of a woman's vagina, as I said earlier, a new vagina can be formed with grafts of skin and muscle. In most cases a vaginal reconstruction is performed at the time of cancer surgery. Until recently, the most widely accepted way to rebuild the vagina was to take flaps of tissue from both inner thighs. More and more, however, doctors have begun using a technique that requires a wedge of skin and muscle from the abdomen, which is then fashioned into an inverted tube. The blood vessels and nerves remain attached to their original site, and the tube is sewn into the area where the vagina has been removed. When the new vagina heals, it is similar in size and shape to the original, and a small scar on the abdomen remains.

Though such a reconstruction does not damage the nerves that control a woman's genital feeling or orgasm, she may need to use a water-soluble lubricant like Astroglide to make intercourse more comfortable. While some survivors with reconstructed vaginas report altered or diminished vaginal sensation, most are gratified that they are able to remain sexually active.

After surgery to create a "neovagina" or following radiation, a woman will be advised to use a special form or mold called a stent, which is worn inside the vagina to keep it stretched out. At first the stent must be used at all times. Then it is worn for most of the night for several months after surgery. After the initial phase of healing, about six to ten weeks, regular sexual intercourse (twice a week) or use of the stent for ten minutes daily is usually enough to keep the vagina open. However, without dilation, the vagina will shrink or scar shut.

Because the new vagina has no way of cleansing itself, your doctor may recommend that after sex you douche with a gentle solution of water and vinegar to prevent discharge and odor. You may also notice some minor bleeding or "spotting" after intercourse, which generally is no cause for alarm. However, if bleeding persists or becomes heavier, contact your doctor immediately.

Vulvectomy

Thanks to new techniques in surgery, a vulvectomy (the treatment for vulvar cancer) is no longer as mutilating and sexually disabling as it was in the past. Nowadays doctors usually are able to preserve the clitoris and replace the diseased vulva with an area of skin taken from the crease of the buttocks. Once the incisions have healed, the look and feel of the genital area is much as it was before. However, because the lymph nodes are also removed, there may be a problem with lymphedema.

Recently I performed such an operation on a stunningly beautiful lawyer named Suzanne, who first came to see me complaining of bumps and sores along the lips outside her vagina. First concerned about ridding herself of cancer, Suzanne then expressed fears about her ability to have intercourse and orgasm. She was forty years old and had enjoyed a monogamous lesbian relationship for the last twelve years. I told her that after four to six weeks of healing, she might notice a strange kind of numbness or tingling around the lips to her vagina, but because I had not removed her clitoris, she'd still be able to reach orgasm as she had before.

Unfortunately, in some forms of progressive vulvar cancer the clitoris may be lost, making it impossible for these women to experience full arousal and orgasm. But some form of pleasure is still possible. Massage or kissing, fondling, stroking, or other kinds of touching that bring the woman into physical contact with her loved one is important. It lets her know she is still desired and wanted on an intimate level.

Vaginal Stenosis

After radiation to the pelvis, a thinning out of the vaginal walls may occur. This condition, known as vaginal stenosis, can cause the vagina to stick shut and scar over, resulting in a permanent shortening of the vaginal canal. When this happens intercourse is not only painful and usually impossible, but a physician may have difficulty inserting a speculum into the vaginal canal to examine a woman's cervix for signs of recurrence.

To avoid these problems, many women are advised to use vaginal dilators, plastic or rubber tubes that "dilate" or stretch out the vagina and keep scar tissue from tightening the canal after radiation. They are not painful and feel much like putting in a large tampon for several minutes each day.

Nevertheless, the first time survivors see a dilator they either gasp with horror or giggle. Still, unless a woman plans to have intercourse on a nightly basis, these devices are the only way to assure she'll be able to have intercourse at all. Depending on the severity of a woman's vaginal stenosis, I usually recommend using a dilator three times a week for ten minutes. Your doctor may suggest a certain way to use your equipment, but generally I tell patients to pick a time of the day when they won't be disturbed for fifteen minutes. Once they have lubricated their device with a water-soluble gel, they should lie down and gently slip the dilator into their vagina. If their vagina feels tight, they should hold the dilator still while they tense and relax their vaginal muscles. They may need to repeat this squeezing exercise several times before the dilator is fully inserted. Once in place, some survivors pass the time by reading, chatting on the telephone, or simply taking a short nap. If it slips out, gently push it back into the vagina. After ten minutes it can be removed and rinsed off with mild soap and water.

At first you may feel a bit hesitant using a dilator, wondering if it is somewhat the same as masturbation. Though sexual pleasure is not its purpose, some women choose to combine this regular stretching of their vagina with sexual pleasure. On occasion, some of my patients have asked if they might substitute a dildo, preferring its contour and softness to the rigid, unnatural look of a dilator. Generally I have no objection. Why not get the fringe benefit of arousal? as one cervical cancer survivor once admitted.

Several months ago a seventy-eight-year-old widow named Ida told me how she'd gone in search of a dildo at a notorious sex shop in New York City. "That dilator you gave me was so clinical looking," she explained. "This friend from my support group told me about a strange little store in Greenwich Village where I could get something better. But do you think it's safe?"

Of course, I told Ida, trying to muffle a laugh as she proudly placed her new purchase on my desk. I could only imagine what the experience must have been like for her. She had probably never seen an X-rated movie in her life, let alone shopped amid the pornographic paraphernalia of New York's Pink Pussycat. But I had to hand it to her. Nothing was going to stop this vibrant little grandmother from keeping her sex life alive.

When Pain Is a Problem

Continued sexual activity is important not only for the emotional well-being of a relationship, but also for the maintenance of proper vaginal health. Regular intercourse at least twice a week serves to stretch a woman's vaginal muscles and toughen up the lining of her canal. But often women experience some discomfort when they first resume having sex. This is usually related to changes in the vagina's size or inability to lubricate itself as a result of pelvic surgery, radiation, or treatment that affects a woman's hormones.

When a woman loses her ovaries to cancer or receives chemotherapy or radiation to her pelvis, she may experience a painful dryness in her genitals, known as vaginal atrophy. Taking tamoxifen can have a similar effect. The lips of her vulva remain dry, and she may develop a particularly sore spot on the outside of her vagina, often between the anus and the vaginal opening, which becomes cracked and tender. Without proper lubrication, the act of thrusting during intercourse can cause tears and sores on the inside of the vaginal canal. If a woman expects to feel pain during sex, she may involuntarily contract her vaginal muscles in anticipation of that pain, a condition known as vaginismus. When her partner tries to push his penis into the vagina, her muscles will spasm shut, increasing the woman's discomfort and lessening her sexual desire.

Estrogen replacement therapy in the form of cream, patches, or pills is often effective for restoring a woman's ability to lubricate and thicken the walls of her vagina. However, the safety of this treatment remains controversial for use in cases of hormonally related cancer of the breast or uterus. For my own patients, I advise against it.

Nevertheless, there are alternatives to solve the problem of vaginal dryness, providing a couple has patience and is willing to make some adjustments in the way they have sex. Many artificial lubricants on the market are successful for restoring moisture in the vagina and can be inserted before sex. Another product, Replens, forms a barrier of synthetic mucus in the vagina that serves as a membrane, providing an extra layer of thickness. It also restores the vagina to a more normal pH, which can prevent bothersome yeast infections.

You may need to try several products before you find one that works for you. You may even need to try several in combination. You may want to try a lubricant like Astroglide, putting a dab's worth on your partner's penis as part of foreplay. This will also help with his erection. Before sex, put a teaspoon's worth on your finger and insert it gently into your vagina. Alternatively, you may prefer a product called Lubrin, which comes in the form of vaginal suppositories. If you try Replens, use it on a Monday, Wednesday, and Friday, unrelated to intercourse. Since most people have a weekend pattern of having sex, enough will have built up by Friday to give you a good barrier of protection.

Since it's common for men to become aroused faster than women, you may need to convey to your partner that you need some time to get to his level of excitement. The areas of a woman's genitals that are most sensitive to touch are the clitoris and inner lips. Like a penis, the clitoris has a head and a shaft and sends messages of pleasure to the brain when it is stroked. Stroking or touching close to, but not on, the head of the clitoris can increase a woman's arousal. A woman may also want to take her partner's penis and stimulate herself.

If pain still remains a problem, switching positions can help. The female superior position, with the woman on top, allows the woman to take more control. Then, if fast or deep thrusting hurts, she can make the movements less deep or slow them down. Another good position is for couples to lie on their sides, either with the man behind the woman, like spoons, or face-to-face. This way you can guide your partner's hands to caress areas of your genitals that feel pleasure and lead him away from areas that may be sore or painful. If intercourse lasts more than ten or fifteen minutes or you have sex more than once, you may need to stop briefly to smooth on some extra lubricant.

Sometimes a shortening of the vagina due to surgery or scarring from radiation can cause pain during intercourse. A couple may need to try different positions to avoid discomfort. Elevating the woman's buttocks with pillows can change the angle of the partner's penis to a more pleasurable position. Or a woman may want to use lubrication on her thighs and keep them shut together to give a sense of a deeper vagina.

However, if pain or burning persists during intercourse, it could be a sign of vaginal infection. Normally a host of bacteria live in the vagina. Cancer therapy can lower your immunity to infection, allowing the more harmful forms of bacteria and fungi to flourish. Check with your doctor. She'll be able to tell you right away if you have moniliasis or some other common form of vaginitis, which are easily treatable with antibiotics.

Sex with a Stoma

No matter how positive a survivor is about recapturing a healthy sexual relationship, facing the practical aspects of dealing with a stoma can have a devastating effect on her self-esteem, disrupting any image she had of herself as attractive and sexual. Let's be honest: stomas are foul smelling and make funny, embarrassing sounds. Many of my patients have found that in order to get over the embarrassment of having one, they have to keep their sense of humor and rely heavily on the support and sensitivity of their partner. One fifty-six-year-old music teacher overcame her initial difficulties by giving her appliance the pet name Puff: "At first, when we tried to have sex, the stoma kept leaking. I was ready to give up hope, but then my husband made a joke by singing the magic dragon song, and he sounded so funny that laughing became a part of our foreplay."

When a woman has a colostomy, she and her husband may have

to plan ahead a bit to avoid unexpected mishaps. To start with, empty your stoma appliance before sex and check the seal before lovemaking. It is also wise to avoid certain foods that day to limit the amount of gas or strong odors. If a leakage does occur during sex, try to laugh it off. You can always jump into the shower with your partner and try again.

To reduce rubbing against the appliance, choose sexual positions that keep your partner's weight off the appliance, or try putting a small pillow above the ostomy. If you or your partner feel uncomfortable exposing the appliance during sex, you may want to purchase a pouch cover that looks less "medical" or wear underwear with the crotch cut out. Some women prefer to tuck the appliance into a wide sash around their waist to keep it out of the way or tape it to their body to keep it from flapping.

Easing into Sex

Every couple feels a bit of apprehension when they decide to resume having sex. A husband may be fearful of hurting his wife, and she may be a bit nervous about how sex will feel. Instead of leaping straight into intercourse, I advise most couples to start off gradually. Pick a time when you won't be interrupted, and enjoy the luxury of each other's company. Soak in a warm bath together, listen to music, light scented candles, or do anything else that relaxes you. Then ease into bed and begin by gently touching and caressing each other's bodies. Sex should be reintroduced as a calming and nondemanding experience, letting a couple rediscover slowly which areas of the woman's body remain sexually sensitive and what areas may feel unpleasant to the touch. It is not important to get sexually excited. If you agree on these goals beforehand, the touching should not be frustrating. Instead, this initial "relearning" session should take away the anxiety and pressure of being close again.

Try to express your desires in a positive way. For instance, "That feels good, but touch it a bit more gently," instead of "Stop it, you're hurting me!" Regardless of your physical problems or medical history, some form of pleasure from sexual touching will always be possible. After a session or two of stroking, many couples progress to genital stroking or oral sex until each partner learns the kinds of touches that bring the other to a higher state of arousal. Because few cancer treatments damage the nerves and muscles responsible for orgasm, a woman can generally be satisfied by having her clitoris stimulated manually or during oral sex. The breasts and nipples are also sources of sexual pleasure for many women. Touching the breasts is a common part of foreplay in our culture. A few women can reach orgasm just from stroking their breasts. For many others, breast stimulation adds to sexual excitement.

If cancer has taken away one of your breasts, you may fear your ability to be stimulated is lost as well. While some women still enjoy being touched around the area of the healed scar, others dislike being stroked there at all and may no longer even enjoy having her partner touch the remaining breast and nipple. You'll have to find your own comfort zone. Some women who have had a mastectomy feel less self-conscious when they place a pillow over the site of surgery or assume positions that make the scar less visible. Others who have stiffness or lymphedema prefer to avoid positions where weight rests on the chest or arm. It may take some time to find a sexual style that works best for both of you, so try to be patient and keep your sense of humor. Once you feel ready, you can begin intercourse.

Redefining Sex

Although cancer doesn't usually destroy the ability to function sexually, it can easily inhibit your sex life. Fatigue, pain, and depression in general can put a damper on your libido. Some chemotherapy drugs may temporarily depress your sex drive. And surgery may leave you limited in the way you perform.

Unfortunately, many couples have a narrow definition of what is "normal" in sex. If both partners cannot reach orgasm while the man's penis is in the woman's vagina, they feel cheated. But there are many other ways of expressing your sexuality besides the act of sexual intercourse. Hugging, cuddling, stroking, massaging, kissing, or verbally expressing love are all expressions of human sensuality. Masturbation can also be a gratifying and acceptable means of sexual pleasure. Though it still carries a stigma for some women, others find that self-stimulation can help maintain their ability to achieve orgasm, increase their sexual drive, and make them feel better in general. However, masturbation is no substitute for sharing with a loving, caring partner.

Homosexuality is also part of the normal range of human sexual behavior, and I often encourage lesbian partners to discuss with me their concerns about sexuality and intimacy, particularly since the literature about homosexual sex after cancer is virtually nil.

Most survivors who were able to achieve orgasm before cancer treatment are still able to do so after treatment. Some will get aroused as easily as they ever did, while others may need some practice. If you're still having trouble, you may need to try something new to push you over the edge of excitement. Different techniques like oral sex or using a vibrator on your genitals may help.

But whatever you try, don't let yourself be tempted by some unproven curative advertised in the back of a magazine. Ginseng, Spanish fly, oysters, rhinoceros horn powder—none of these so-called aphrodisiacs work, and pursuing such useless treatments not only wastes your time and money, but also may be harmful to your health. If you and your partner have serious concerns about your sex life, speak with your oncologist or gynecologist. Ideally, she can suggest a specialist in sexual problems who can help you and your partner develop better communication and more enjoyment of touching. If your partner resists seeing such a counselor, perhaps your doctor can speak with him privately and help to get him more involved.

Sex and the Single Survivor

When you're in a long-term relationship, concerns and conflicts about sexuality are never easy. If you're single and have to face the dating scene, they can seem almost impossible. How do you tell a new boyfriend that you've had cancer? Is it best to wait until you feel a sense of trust and caring from him—or should you tell him on the first date so your feelings aren't hurt later on? What if things are moving more quickly? How do you broach the entire issue of sex when you've lost a breast, or wear an ostomy, or have problems with vaginal lubrication? Should you tell him one breast isn't real? If you have hopes to marry or to remarry, you may even question whether to involve a new lover in a future that still seems shaky.

These are difficult issues with uncertain answers. Embarrassment about her altered body, fear that her sexual interest and response may have decreased, and a sense of somehow being devalued because of infertility can interfere with a woman's openness to pursue new involvements. Anticipating rejection if she reveals her history of cancer, a survivor may even avoid opportunities to develop new love relationships.

Gwen, now twenty-five, developed Hodgkin's lymphoma when she was only thirteen, requiring surgeons to make a nine-inch incision down her torso to remove her spleen and lymph nodes. "When I was growing up, I always wore bathing suits that covered my scar, and I learned to wear blouses I could tuck in my pants. Most of my high school friends knew what I'd been through and were good about never teasing me. But when I got to college and started dating a new group of guys, there were always questions. Sometimes I told them right away and sometimes I waited, hoping they'd understand. But whenever I told them I had cancer, the tenor of the relationship always changed."

As women like Gwen come to realize, there will always be men who reject you because of cancer. It's a hard issue to grasp, especially when you're just starting to know someone. But everyone gets rejected sometimes—whether they had cancer or not—and it may have more to do with your lack of shared interests, or your inability to communicate well, than about your having once had a deadly disease.

Granted, you can always stay home and never reach out for companionship or love. But in doing so, you may never meet that special man who will cherish and care for you in spite of cancer. Don't lose sight of the fact that you're quite an extraordinary woman, who's endured a life-threatening situation and survived. Chances are there's a man out there who will look at your courage, your strength to rebound from hardship, and admire and love you for that alone.

Diane, forty-three, discovered she had breast cancer three months after her divorce. She got a reconstruction and was just back on her feet when cancer struck again in her other breast. Unfortunately her second reconstruction didn't turn out as successfully as the first. "There was puckering from the scar tissue, and they didn't look entirely even. But I decided if that's what a guy is really concerned about, then I'm not interested in pursuing a relationship with him. Cancer changed the way I think about life, and I want to find a man for whom beauty is more than skin deep."

There are no strict rules about how to handle relationships when you've had cancer. But if you find you're feeling shy about meeting new people, ask a trusted friend to take the role of a new dating partner and rehearse what you'd like to say. Have her react in a way that you fear the most, then practice your response. When you feel confidence in yourself and seem able to handle rejection, you're ready to take the plunge. It won't always be easy. The dating scene never is. But as long as you view it as a learning experience and not a trauma to be endured, you're likely to find some measure of success.

Sex and the Older Woman

Slowly, society is coming to accept the idea that older women still enjoy active sex lives. A woman may be past her prime, but this doesn't mean her need and desire for intimacy are on the wane. Recent research confirms that middle-aged and older women retain their sexual responsiveness. In one report, which surveyed eight hundred adults between the ages of sixty and ninety, a large number reported that sex was better than ever. Many women said their orgasms were even more intense than in their youth and revealed they experimented with various positions and forms of stimulation to increase their sexual enjoyment. Age alone was not enough to eliminate interest and pleasure for most respondents. In fact, many noted that giving pleasure rather than aiming for orgasm relieved them of the pressure to perform and freed them to experience the joy of relating.

But when an older woman survives cancer, she may find herself wondering if sex is still safe, let alone possible. Decreased vaginal lubrication can make lovemaking difficult and possibly painful. Physical scars may make her feel unappealing and untouchable. And if she or her partner suffer from another medical condition like high blood pressure, arthritis, or diabetes, there might be other sexual problems to contend with.

Though women should directly discuss their concerns with their partner, many are reluctant to bring up the subject of sex. It's not something most older women feel comfortable discussing. They may think that vaginal intercourse is the only legitimate form of sex and that other intimate exchanges such as oral sex, manual stimulation, or masturbation are indecent. But as I try to tell my older patients, physical and emotional intimacy with those you love is a very important element for living a quality life. Sexual activity can encompass more than just intercourse. Touching, laughing, caring, and playing are all expressions of human sensuality. These needs never change and do not require the perfect body of youth to be fulfilled. Sexual intercourse may not even be a part of lovemaking eventually. What is important is the intimate relationship between partners.

If you're worried about sex, you should speak with your physician. She's there to counsel and treat you for *any* problems you may be having. She may suggest changing your sexual routines: intimacy is often more successful and gratifying for older couples in the morning, when they have more energy, than at night. Taking a warm bath can often relieve pain stemming from stiffness of the joints. Engaging in sexual activities other than intercourse can help to alleviate anxiety and enable older people to better enjoy their sexual relations.

But above all, remember: It is normal to enjoy and be interested in sex throughout your life. Having cancer may change the way you have sex, but it doesn't have to stop you from enjoying the pleasures of intimacy, no matter what your age or physical limitations.

Seven

THE ROAD TO MOTHERHOOD

Before cancer, Leslie and her husband, Tom, had always taken for granted that they would have children. Like many young couples, they spent the first years of their marriage establishing their careers and building a nest egg so that one day they could settle down in a house of their own to raise a family.

"Money was tight at first, but eventually we saved enough to buy the perfect little cottage," recalls Leslie, a New York architect. "There was an extra bedroom just big enough for my drafting table and a crib. In another couple of months, we were going to start our family."

But then, at thirty-four, Leslie got ovarian cancer. First there was surgery, then chemotherapy to ward off the spread of disease. Days of enduring sickness stretched into months of uncommon strength and courage, taking away the couple's ordinary life and happiness.

Nearly one year following chemotherapy, Leslie was ready to begin rebuilding her life. On a Friday afternoon in July, she and Tom met with me in my office, tensely gripping each other's hands. "I have terrific news," I told her. "The tests show no new sign of disease."

Leslie was thirty-five. Alive. Cancer-free. "Whatever you did before, you can do again," I reassured her. "You can get your life back to normal."

"But, a baby," she said, her eyes welling up with tears. "Can I still have a baby?"

Surviving cancer clearly complicates the issue of pregnancy, but it doesn't always mean an end to what is for many women a lifelong goal. More and more women are having children after cancer. But the decision to do so must be undertaken with a great deal of forethought and consideration. The experience of battling and triumphing over cancer heightens every aspect of pregnancy—the risks, the emotions, the fears, and the expectations. Before a survivor can approach such a monumental life choice, she and her partner need to have a firm grasp of the medical information available and a clear understanding of how it relates to her own particular history of cancer.

Just a few decades ago it was rare to hear of a woman becoming pregnant after cancer. Cancer seemed to be an illness a woman developed in middle age or old age, long after her childbearing years were over. In our parents' day, most women were in their twenties when they bore children; the threat of cancer interfering with motherhood was, if anything, a distant and abstract notion.

Today the proportion of women under forty who develop and survive cancer is rising steadily. Dramatic medical advances in treatment and cure rates are allowing women with cancer to live longer than ever before. The American Cancer Society predicts that by the year 2000 more than five million women will have won the battle against this dread disease, creating a significant population of survivors who want to become pregnant.

But after cancer, the road to motherhood may not be easy. Deciding to have a child brings up a host of doubts and fears you will want to discuss with your doctor. Has cancer affected my ability to get pregnant? Will the treatments I've had complicate my pregnancy or cause birth defects? Will getting pregnant make my cancer come back? Will I be able to see my child grow up? And perhaps the most vexing question of all: Will the child I bear end up getting my disease?

Pregnancy after cancer is certainly not a choice for every woman, and answers to these critical questions are not always clear-cut and decisive. A couple must balance the risks of having children against their own unique set of needs and priorities. After speaking with Leslie and Tom about their desire for a child, Leslie admitted to me: "What I'm really trying to do is stave off the inevitable, which is death. When I tell you I want a child, what I'm really saying is, 'I don't want to die.'"

This desire is really the same for *any* woman and man who want to continue the chain of life in their children and on through future generations. Having a child can be a way of reaching toward immortality, of letting a piece of you live on for posterity. But the cancer survivor may also find that it helps her feel as though she's once again moving within the natural cycle of life. Knowing that a life is growing inside gives many women a confidence about their restored health and self-identity, adding profound meaning to the new beginning mother and child share together.

Of course, not all survivors will be able to conceive or bear children. But that doesn't mean they cannot experience the joys, challenges, and fulfillment of motherhood. Today's burgeoning array of assisted reproductive technologies now give many survivors choices and possibilities where before there were none. Adoption, stepparenting, and foster parenting also allow survivors a chance at motherhood and a way to make their own contribution to the upbringing of a child.

Last year, after one of my cervical cancer patients adopted a four-year-old boy with Down's syndrome, she wrote to me about her decision: "Surviving cancer taught me that hell has an exit, and that nothing is impossible. I needed to show this to a child who had always thought there would never be a mother to love him. When I brought Ryan home, it seemed as if we were destined to be a family all along."

Making the Decision

Motherhood after cancer is clearly possible for many survivors, but it is not a decision to enter into lightly. To first confirm whether you will be able to carry a child—as well as how safe it will be to do so—these four important factors must be considered:

> How old are you?
> What kind of cancer did you have?
> What kind of surgery and/or treatment did you receive?
> How long has it been since treatment ended
>   and you have been disease-free?

Research has shown that if a woman under forty wants to get pregnant after cancer, most of the time she can, providing, of course, that her reproductive organs are intact and functioning and any chemotherapy or radiation treatments she received did not disrupt her menstrual periods or scar her reproductive tract to prevent the normal cycle of eggs from descending the fallopian tubes.

You should know, however, that pregnancy itself may have risks. Though many potential problems can be eliminated through careful monitoring and treatment, there is always the chance for problems. Chemotherapy and radiation can weaken the function of certain critical organs like the heart, lungs, and kidneys. During pregnancy and labor, these organs may be stressed further to take care of the needs of both mother and baby. Before getting pregnant, discuss with your doctor whether pregnancy will jeopardize your health in any way.

You also should consider carefully if any physical limitations caused by cancer treatment will affect your ability to care for a child. Several chapters ago I mentioned how one of my patients needed a special sling to hold her baby because the neuropathy in her hands sometimes caused her to jerk uncontrollably. A seemingly small disability from cancer can be magnified by the day-to-day rigors of motherhood: constantly lifting and carrying a youngster, twisting off caps on baby food jars and bottles, pushing a stroller, diapering, and, of course, those endless middle-of-the-night feedings. Raising a child is an awesome responsibility, whether you've had cancer or not. Before making the decision, you need to acknowledge the potential stumbling blocks and make certain you have a realistic view of what life with a child will really be like.

If you opt to go ahead, gather up as much information as you can about your medical history and that of your partner. Make a list of all the diagnoses, surgeries, and treatments you received, along with the dosages and administration dates. Then find yourself an obstetrician/gynecologist who will work in close conjunction with the oncologist who treated your cancer, as well as with other members of the medical team that got you through your illness.

You'll need to give your doctors a detailed history of your attempts to become pregnant, both before and since cancer. If you had trouble conceiving before cancer, both you and your partner may want to consult a fertility specialist trained in reproductive endocrinology and add him or her to your medical team.

Remember that medical opinions about having children after cancer differ widely; you may receive very disparate responses from doctors you speak with—ranging from encouraging to disparaging. You and your partner should feel free to consult several doctors about your chances of delivering a healthy baby, as well as how safe it will be for you to do so. Build a consensus of the best medical advice available. If you and your partner still wish to become parents, be sure to choose a doctor who realistically assesses your medical history and informs you honestly about the risks involved—but who will be absolutely supportive about helping you reach your goal. You will both need a doctor you can rely on, someone you feel is one hundred percent on your side.

To help you have a clearer understanding of what issues you may confront, let's now explore the latest evidence on how cancer affects a woman's prospects for having children.

A Question of Fertility

When cancer strikes a woman's uterus, ovaries, cervix, or part of her lower bowel, doctors may be forced to remove important reproductive systems that could preclude her from conceiving or bearing children. Even when the organs necessary to reproduction are left in place, pelvic surgery can sometimes cause adhesions or scarring of the fallopian tubes or abdominal cavity that may disrupt a woman's fertility.

What is more, chemotherapy may also thwart a woman's ability to conceive by interfering with her body's production of hormones and interrupting her monthly cycle, resulting in amenorrhea (suppressed menstrual periods) or premature menopause. Though these effects may be only temporary, the more aggressive and long term chemotherapy is, the higher the risk for permanent ovarian failure.

Often, a woman's age at time of treatment will influence whether or not her reproductive system will bounce back after chemotherapy. Medical evidence shows that women over forty frequently enter menopause after chemotherapy, whereas younger women usually resume menstruation after treatment, without any effect on their ability to conceive. Numerous studies have documented successful pregnancies in survivors of lymphatic cancers, leukemia, and malignant germ cell tumors of one ovary after treatment with combination chemotherapy. While alkylating drugs like Alkeran and Cytoxan are most likely to affect fertility, research shows a woman still has a good chance of becoming pregnant if she was under forty at the time of treatment. Research shows that approximately 40 to 50 percent of women treated with combination chemotherapy, particularly MOPP (Mustargen, Oncovin, Procarbazine, Prednisone) or related regimens, lose their periods. For women over thirty-nine, the loss of periods was permanent; in women younger than thirty-five, the ovaries resumed function, with the data suggesting that for the five to ten years following therapy, their periods would continue. But only with continued long-term follow-up of survivors will we be able to determine the risk of premature ovarian failure and early menopause.

Radiation to the pelvis most often results in infertility due to its effects on the ovaries and the uterus. Radiation causes premature ovarian failure and scars the lining of the uterus or fallopian tubes. Fortunately oncologists are now developing innovative techniques for protecting a woman's ovaries prior to treatment. Recently I operated on a thirty-three-year-old woman named Delia with adenocarcinoma of the cervix. She had gone to her gynecologist for some standard tests before trying to get pregnant, but instead her doctor discovered a huge lesion at the mouth of her uterus, requiring a hysterectomy and radiation therapy. Before I removed her uterus, I repositioned her ovaries to waist level, outside the area that would be irradiated. Though she is no longer able to bear a child, Delia still hopes that one day she'll have eggs extracted from her ovaries and have them fertilized by her husband's sperm. She'll then be able to "borrow" a uterus—most likely that of her sister—to have a child that is biologically her own.

Hope for the Infertile

"Having children was something I had always wanted to do, to experience the growth of life inside me. When cancer took this dream away, it felt like I had lost two lives—mine and the one I may have had one day," says Lisa, thirty-eight, a breast cancer survivor who received such toxic doses of chemotherapy that it wiped out her ability to get pregnant.

Infertility is one of the most tragic complications of cancer therapy. It can be devastating to learn that in the battle to sustain life, your potential to create a new human being has been lost. Thousands of cancer survivors face this problem each year.

Fortunately there is hope. As my patient Delia's story illustrates, many new possibilities are available for survivors left sterile or unable physically to bear a child. Remarkable advances in reproductive technology such as in vitro fertilization, embryo transfer, and surrogate wombs now allow survivors and their partners the option to have children who are genetically their own.

But before a couple opts to try one of these newer procedures, they should understand the emotional and financial price. Generally, assisted reproductive technology is invasive, time-consuming, and often painful emotionally. And at best, a survivor's chances of getting pregnant are only one out of four. Studies show that the stress and emotional commitment involved can be so trying that half of the couples who don't get pregnant end up divorced a year after treatment.

To further complicate the picture, the average cost of one of these new technologies is between $6,000 and $20,000 per try, depending on the type of procedure, the clinic used, and the clinic's geographical location. So far, only ten states—Arkansas, California, Connecticut, Hawaii, Illinois, Maryland, Massachusetts, Rhode Island, New York, and Texas—require health insurance companies to either offer or cover the costs of infertility treatment.

Of the estimated three hundred assisted-fertility clinics operating nationwide, all are required by federal law to report their success rate uniformly, so that couples can sort through their widely competing claims. No rules specify whom clinics can treat by age, marital status, or health history. If you and your partner still think you'd like to try for a child with assisted reproductive technology, first consult with your oncologist and gynecologist. They can outline the risks of pregnancy, labor, and delivery as well as the dangers associated with multiple gestation, the incidence of premature delivery, and other neonatal problems associated with some of these reproductive technologies.

In Vitro Fertilization (IVF)

In vitro fertilization, or artificial conception, is the cornerstone for many of the newer reproductive technologies and the procedure of choice when surgical scarring or infection prevents an egg from traveling through the fallopian tubes into the uterus. During IVF, several eggs are removed from a woman's ovaries and mixed with a sample of her partner's sperm. (In the beginning, test tubes were used for insemination—hence the term *test-tube baby*—but these days laboratory dishes are used instead.) Two or three days later the fertilized embryos are transferred through the vagina into the woman's uterus.

The advantages of IVF are that fertilization can be confirmed and the quality of the resulting embryos can be assessed for chromosomal damage before implantation. However, the chance that IVF will result in a successful pregnancy is still only about 20 percent. Experts have learned that the best way to beat these odds is to fertilize and implant several embryos simultaneously. Typically, doctors achieve this by giving the mother hormones that cause her to superovulate, or produce more than one egg at a time. The more embryos transferred, the greater the likelihood of pregnancy.

But hormone treatments harbor their own risks: if multiple embryos succeed in gestating, a woman may find herself at high risk for miscarriage or premature delivery. The drugs themselves are also known to produce uncomfortable side effects ranging from headaches and weight gain to mood swings, irritability, and depression. Still worse, a 1993 study reported that infertile women who used fertility drugs and did not become pregnant had a significantly increased risk of developing ovarian cancer. Although the study was highly criticized for flaws in its methodology, further research has shown a similar link between fertility drugs and cancer. More data is needed to confirm this association, but women who take these drugs need to be aware of the potential risk and to inform their oncologist and gynecologist of this drug history.

Gamete Intrafallopian Transfer (GIFT)

A GIFT procedure involves retrieving eggs and placing them directly into a woman's fallopian tubes with a large number of her partner's sperm. Before transfer, the eggs are analyzed quickly under a microscope to select the ones most likely to be fertilized. These are then put into a fallopian tube, which is thought to be a better site for fertilization to occur. However, there is no guarantee that this will happen or, if it does, that implantation to the uterus will be successful.

Zygote Intrafallopian Transfer (ZIFT)

A ZIFT procedure involves retrieving and inseminating eggs as they are for IVF. The zygote (the fertilized embryo that has not yet divided) is placed in the fallopian tube one or two days after retrieval. ZIFT has the advantages of both IVF and GIFT: fertilization can be determined, and the fallopian tube is used as an incubator. There are also disadvantages, however: the process is more costly and involves two days of procedures (including a laparoscopy), and although fertilization is guaranteed, the quality of the embryo cannot be assured after one day.

Ovum Donation

When cancer treatment causes a woman to stop ovulating, she still has the option of using donated eggs to become pregnant. After finding a willing donor—sometimes the survivor's friend or family member, sometimes a stranger who is paid for her help—doctors prepare both women for the ovum transfer. The donor receives hormonal treatments to increase the number of eggs produced during her menstrual cycle. The survivor gets a different hormonal treatment to prepare her womb for pregnancy. When the donor starts to ovulate, the doctor inserts a needle through her vaginal or abdominal wall to extract eggs from her ovaries. The donor eggs are then combined with sperm from the survivor's partner to create viable embryos. Several of these growing embryos are then inserted vaginally into the prospective mother's womb, in the hope that one will develop.

Studies show that success rates after ovum donation are better than other methods of assisted conception, probably because eggs are usually obtained from young women and possibly because the uterus of the recipient has not been exposed to the hormonal changes induced by fertility drugs.

Nevertheless, pregnancy usually takes more than one try and may end in multiple births. Also, a couple needs to consider the many unresolved legal and social implications surrounding ovum donation. Should the child be told about its genetic mother? Does the donor have legal responsibility to the child? These and other questions will surely arise as the budding technology of ovum donation continues to evolve.

Surrogacy

When a woman loses her uterus or has chemotherapy or radiation that damages her ability to bear children, she still can fulfill her need to have a child by "borrowing" another woman's uterus. Usually such an intimate request is made to a close friend or relative, although paid surrogates are an option, albeit a controversial one.

Two types of surrogacy exist. If a woman's ovaries are still intact and producing healthy eggs, these eggs can be removed and fertilized with her partner's sperm through IVF. The resulting embryo is then transferred to the surrogate's womb and, with luck, carried to term. If a woman has no viable eggs of her own, the surrogate's own eggs are artificially inseminated with sperm from the cancer survivor's partner. In either case, the surrogate then surrenders the baby to the survivor and her husband at birth.

In theory, surrogacy is an easy process. In reality, however, it is fraught with complex and controversial issues. Before a survivor and her partner take any steps to begin the surrogacy process, it is critical they consult a skilled and reputable lawyer. As the Baby M case demonstrated so dramatically, countless legal and ethical questions surround surrogacy, and it is imperative that provisions be made to safeguard the privacy and well-being of the survivor and her family-to-be.

Future Reproductive Techniques

In the future, doctors hope to give women the option of removing their eggs *before* cancer treatment, freezing them safely for use at a later date. Researchers are also experimenting with techniques that would allow women to have strips of their ovaries frozen and put back after treatment was over. One day it too may be feasible to transplant ovaries from aborted fetuses into infertile survivors who no longer can make viable eggs of their own. Doctors already have perfected these methods in laboratory animals, but it remains to be seen if they will be medically successful, let alone ethically acceptable, for use in human beings.

Breast Cancer and Pregnancy

Perhaps the most terrifying fear of any mother—especially one who has lived through cancer—is that she might not live long enough to raise her own children. This is a particularly torturous dilemma for breast cancer survivors who worry that the hormonal surges of pregnancy might trigger a recurrence of their disease. Two years ago the National Cancer Institute reviewed the medical literature on this issue and found no evidence indicating that pregnancy following treatment for breast cancer influences the outcome of the disease. The published reports represent a selected group of women. A favorable outcome may merely represent a sampling bias. However, some data on animals suggest that the level of hormones present in pregnancy may actually have a suppressive effect on tumor growth. This could explain why subsequent pregnancies following breast cancer have not been associated with earlier recurrences or decreased survival. Based on this data, it would appear that choosing to carry a child will *probably not* significantly affect a woman's prognosis.

Still, when a doctor reassures a breast cancer survivor that a pregnancy probably won't influence the course of her disease, it doesn't mean he is able to predict if she will live to see her child through to adulthood. Though a doctor can advise a woman how her individual risk factors *may* impact her chances for recurrent disease, there are no absolute guidelines for women who want a baby after breast cancer. Nor are there guarantees that she will live a long life and see her child grow up to bear children of her own. As a result, each survivor must make her own decision, basing it not only on the medical risks and uncertainties involved, but also on her own medical history, prognosis, and circumstances.

"After losing both my breasts—one to a mastectomy, the other prophylactically—I asked if it was safe to have a baby," says Cynthia, thirty-seven. "Three doctors offered three opinions: Never become pregnant again, because the hormones released during gestation would act like gasoline on a fire if any cancer cells remained; wait at least two years before conceiving; and go ahead, since pregnancy should be as safe for me as for any woman, because I had had no chemotherapy and was node negative—thus, presumably, cancer-free.

"My husband and I were confused but decided to try to conceive. My daughter, Olivia, now four, was the result, and those of us who love her know what a good decision that was."

Most doctors recommend a two- to three-year wait after treatment before trying to get pregnant. This waiting period is based on the fact that recurrence peaks in the first two years. Approximately one-third of the population at risk will have recurrences during the first three years. However, this waiting period may be inappropriate for women who had small, node-negative tumors. Almost 85 percent of women with small, localized breast cancer can expect to live ten years or more.

For women with positive nodes, the situation is less clear. When cancer invades the lymph nodes, a woman's chances of five-year survival drop to 30 to 60 percent, depending on the number of nodes involved. It's believed that the longer a survivor goes without recurrence of her disease, the better her long-term chances for survival. Even so, the survival curves continue to fall—even at ten years the curve has not plateaued. For women with widely metastatic or recurrent disease, pregnancy should not be considered because of the poor prognosis and need for ongoing treatment.

There may also be other characteristics about your breast cancer that will influence your risks for recurrence. When you discuss getting pregnant with your doctor, be sure to get answers to these important questions:

- *What was the size of my breast tumor?* Generally, a lesion smaller than two centimeters is referred to as an "early stage" breast cancer and has a lesser chance of spreading to outlying organs and tissue than one that is larger than two centimeters. The smaller the tumor, the greater a woman's chances to survive five years or more.
- *Did my tumor invade nearby lymph nodes?* The risk of breast cancer recurrence is greatest during the first two years after treatment and

occurs more often in women with positive lymph node involvement. The number of involved lymph nodes is also important—more than four carries a high risk of recurrence.

• *What was my tumor's estrogen and progesterone receptor status?* If a woman's tumor receptors were estrogen positive and progesterone positive, her outlook for long-term survival is usually good. If she was estrogen positive but progesterone negative, she is still better off than having both receptors negative.

Also check with your physician to see if the following oncogene research tests were performed on your tumor; though still considered "investigational," they may supply useful information to predict your overall chance for recurrence:

• *Was my tumor HER-2/neu positive?* Studies show that breast tumors that are positive for HER-2/neu usually recur within two years of diagnosis.
• *What was the "ploidy" of my tumor?* Cancer with a genetic characteristic known as "aneuploid" usually carries a higher risk of recurrence than one with its "diploid" counterpart.
• *Did my tumor express epidermal growth factor?* When a woman's breast tumor expresses an epidermal growth factor, her chances of recurrence are generally higher.

Together with your oncologist and obstetrician/gynecologist, you can make a decision that's right for you. The decision will be based on the prognosis of your particular type of tumor, the time elapsed since your cancer was treated, and your ability to integrate the care of a child into your life and that of your family.

Cancer's Genetic Legacy

When a cancer survivor contemplates having a child, one of her chief concerns is whether her child will be born genetically sound.

Once again, there are no guarantees. The risk of congenital abnormalities can occur in *any* pregnancy. Though the numbers of patients available for study are still small, most evidence seems to show that children born to women treated with chemotherapy have no increased incidence of birth defects or genetic malformations. However, a few reports cite an 8 to 10 percent increased incidence of congenital anomalies. Women treated with both chemotherapy and radiation may have a greater chance of miscarriage or fetal abnormality. Though an overall review of the published data is reassuring, more studies carried out over many years will be required before the true risks to subsequent generations are known.

In a manner, this allays some women's fears. Yet there is always the nagging worry that by having children, a survivor will inadvertently pass along a genetic predisposition for cancer. Doctors now know that certain types of cancer—uterine, breast, ovary, and colon—can be inherited. But it still remains a mystery why most of the women affected by these diseases have no family history. Until researchers can figure out why, a cancer survivor must assume that if she has children, she may be passing along a potential legacy for her disease. Even if there is no family history for cancer in her background, a survivor needs to realize that once she developed cancer, she *became* the family history.

This doesn't mean your children will inevitably get cancer. No one can say with absolute certainty who will get any disease. But researchers have found that when cancer is hereditary, the risk of developing it is enormous. Approximately 5 percent of women with breast cancer inherit a defective copy of the gene known as BRCA1. When a mother passes this gene to her daughter, she has an 85 percent chance of getting breast cancer during her lifetime!

Though this may make some women hesitant to get pregnant for fear of passing along damaged genetic goods, there is hope. Recently geneticists have also located the specific gene responsible for a relatively common form of colon cancer, and at least one company has announced plans to begin offering testing for genetic cancer risk. Chances are by the time a survivor's child is old enough to develop one of these hereditary cancers, there will be screening techniques to sample their DNA for defective genes and perhaps even therapy to modify those risks.

Until then, however, the best a survivor can do is give her children the gifts of foreknowledge and healthy, cancer-preventing habits they can take into adulthood. By knowing the risks, your daughter (or son) will be able to inform doctors of the family's medical history, so that steps can be taken to screen for any early signs of disease.

Leslie, the ovarian cancer survivor we met at the start of this chapter, has her own mother, Rhoda, to thank for just such a forewarning. Rhoda knew that her grandmother had passed away from a mysterious stomach ailment, so she began asking questions about her family's medical history. She contacted relatives, did some library research, and eventually was able to trace ovarian cancer back to two maternal relatives. There were also multiple cases of colon, endometrial (uterine lining), and breast cancer on her mother's side. When she discussed these findings with her gynecologist, she learned how certain families appear to carry genes that may lead to a hereditary cancer syndrome. One syndrome can cause ovarian cancer; a second, either ovarian or breast cancer; and a third, ovarian, endometrial, colon, and/or prostate cancer in family members who inherit the defective gene. Because there were clusters of all these cancers in her family background—and particularly because they appeared in some relatives under the age of fifty—the risk to Rhoda, her daughter Leslie, and any of their female descendants was probably as high as 50 percent. In these syndromes, *both* sides of the family are important with respect to transmitting inherited disease.

Thus far, cancer has yet to strike Rhoda. But because she knows it may be only a matter of time, she is screened rigorously for the disease every six months. Leslie was also careful to be checked regularly, and it was during one of these biannual checkups that doctors discovered an early tumor on her right ovary.

"I'm alive today because of my mother's efforts," says Leslie, who naturally felt some apprehension on discovering that her remaining ovary still allowed her to have children. "I worried about what I might pass along to my child. But I also saw getting pregnant as a way of reaffirming my own existence. If I didn't have children, I'd always feel I turned a possible risk into a lifelong tragedy."

Making a Genogram

If you suspect that a certain cancer is being passed down through your family, you may want to visit a genetic counselor in your area. Generally a large medical center or teaching hospital will have a cancer-screening program, where a genetic counselor can evaluate your risk and help you determine proper family prevention and care. For gynecologic cancers, a gynecologic oncologist may be your best resource.

Before you go, gather up as much medical information about your family as you can, so you can use it to construct a genogram, or family health tree. Ask your parents and other family members about medical details—names, birth dates, death dates—for relatives on both sides of your family, ideally going back three or four generations.

Your aim is to determine the major illnesses, age at onset, cause of death, and age at death for each of your relatives—especially siblings, parents, aunts, uncles, first cousins, and grandparents. You may need to contact the physician or hospital that treated a relative, then have your own doctor ask for copies of their medical records. Because many Americans are descended from peoples across the world, it may be difficult, even impossible, to obtain certain medical records. It may help if you obtain the pamphlet *Where to Write for Vital Records:* contact the Superintendent of Documents, P.O. Box 371954, Pittsburgh, PA 15250-7954. You also can try contacting the town hall where a relative lived to get copies of their death certificate. But bear in mind that death certificates are often too general or even misleading. For example, the term *carcinomatosis*, which often appears on documents more than twenty years old, indicates widespread cancer without telling where the tumor began.

Even so, it's important to discuss any suspicious findings with an oncologist or genetic counselor. A strong pattern of cancer does *not* mean your children are destined to suffer the disease. But for some women, the very fact that there might be a gene for cancer can help to finalize their decision about pregnancy. I know from a personal standpoint that if I had not gone into premature menopause after chemotherapy, I still would not have had children, mainly because I couldn't bear to think of them getting breast cancer because of me.

On the other hand, there are women like Leslie who choose to go ahead, using the knowledge of their cancer background as an impetus for teaching children good health habits and effective cancer-screening techniques. They see cancer as a disease that needs to be discussed openly within the family, not hidden and suffered in silence as it was in generations gone by.

No one should judge a woman on the basis of whether she's had cancer or not. Nor should they decide for her whether having children is right or wrong. Though surviving cancer may not jibe with society's ideal image of motherhood, the choice is one every woman needs to make on a personal and individual basis with her partner, her doctor, and her conscience. As many cancer survivors learn, being a good mother really has nothing to do with one's health history. It all depends on love and honesty, patience and caring, and above all a woman's complete devotion to another person whose very being affirms the endless possibilities that life has to offer.

Recently I saw this to be true when I attended a function we have at the hospital known as Cancer Survivors Day. Former patients are invited to stand up, introduce themselves, and talk about their accomplishments. As you might imagine, these festivities are always a source of profound inspiration—but this year's event took on a special sweetness when I noticed one of my own patients approach the podium.

"Hi, I'm Leslie," she began, her voice quavering but brimming with joy. "My husband, my mother, and my doctor are here with me today." Silence blanketed the room as everyone anticipated her next words. Finally she took a deep breath and help up the squirming bundle in her arms. "I had ovarian cancer four years ago, and this is Jennifer, my brand-new baby daughter."

Eight

CANCER'S EFFECT ON THE FAMILY

Some time ago, as I was nearing the end of my radiation treatments for breast cancer, my husband suggested we celebrate his birthday by going to the theater. A patient had given him tickets for an Off-Broadway production that we'd heard was a lighthearted comedy about the female bonding experience. Instead the play turned out to be a gripping portrayal of a young woman dying of breast cancer.

At first I thought of leaving the theater. "Haven't we had enough of this damned disease?" I whispered to Sheldon during the first act. But as the play progressed, I found myself drawn to the performance of the woman's husband. His words seemed to echo every family's feelings of loss: the disbelief and denial of his wife's diagnosis, the rage and confusion during her treatment, the anxiety and fear of watching her suffer. In a moving soliloquy toward the end of the play, he expressed how difficult a husband's pain could be, how in listening to the groans of his wife and in ministering to her needs, no one had once acknowledged his own feelings. It was always "How is your wife? How is *she* doing?" But weren't his own fears of being left behind in some way important? Didn't he too deserve some measure of comfort and support during her illness?

When the performance ended, Sheldon and I both sat motionless and quiet. There was no need for words. He, above all others, knew how grueling and debilitating my cancer treatments had been. But until then, I'd been too focused on my disease to acknowledge the emotional misery that he too must have suffered.

After learning you have cancer, your one and only goal becomes survival. In an effort to stay alive, you shut yourself off from the rest of the world and its responsibilities, using every ounce of your energy just to get out of bed and get through treatment. Rarely do you have the will, let alone the desire, to confront the avalanche of emotions that lies behind the supportive smiles of your family and friends. Only when your ordeal has ended and you've achieved remission can you see what a devastating effect the disease has had, not only on yourself, but also on those closest to you.

As survivors, each of us faces a day of reckoning when we must look beyond the circle of cancer and reach out to life: get back in touch with friends, deal with changes and compromises in our daily lives, and relearn how to interact with members of our own family.

But as many of us discover, this is seldom an easy process. Even after the ordeal of treatment, when a woman is declared disease-free, cancer still has a way of disrupting the fragile emotions and relationships within a family. After months spent nursing a loved one through therapy, relatives may be eager to return to the status quo, expecting the survivor promptly to do the same. Or they may react in an opposite manner, going out of their way to overprotect and overindulge the survivor at a time when she's trying to regain her sense of self-esteem and independence.

A husband may begin harboring feelings of resentment and anger when his wife doesn't bounce back as quickly as he anticipated. Or a daughter might pull away and seem distant as a way of protecting herself against the fear of recurrence. Even old friends may stop calling, unsure how to respond.

At the same time, the survivor herself may find it hard to give up the advantages of being a patient and return to the customary demands of life. The sheer weight of resuming her role as the emotional center of her family—of once again becoming the concerned wife, the ever-interested parent, the devoted daughter, or the doting grandparent—can be overwhelming, particularly when these responsibilities take time away from the rest and relaxation she needs to recover.

After cancer, every family experiences a range of conflicting emotions: joy and fear, hopefulness and anxiety, love and anger. There may be difficulty adjusting to new roles and routines, problems helping younger children cope, and stress in learning that cancer may now run in the family.

There is no simple solution to ease this transition from illness to recovery. But when family members are willing to share their feelings with each other and to talk about the disease and the changes it brings, concerns about the future may seem less ominous. Granted, this can be a painful process of discovery. But it can also serve to strengthen the bonds between you and help make life after cancer as rewarding and fulfilling as possible.

Hidden Emotions

When a woman survives cancer, she still must live with the haunting fear that one day her disease might return. It's a terrifying prospect and one that many survivors and their families find too frightening to discuss. Wary of shattering the thin layer of hope that exists, they hide their true feelings and concerns, expressing them instead through more negative emotions like anger and resentment.

When Evelyn, a fifty-six-year-old survivor of ovarian cancer, returned home after surgery, she was unable to tell her husband, Milton, how frightened she still was. Instead she grew irritable and distant when he expected her to join in family activities as she had before her illness. "Doesn't he realize how sick I've been?" she confided to me. When I asked to speak with Milton separately, he also sounded bitter: "How long do I have to wait before her cancer is out of our lives? We used to do things as a family, and now all she wants to do is stay home alone."

Another patient named Carla would get into raging arguments with her husband before each of her follow-up exams for cervical cancer. At our last appointment together, I pointed out that fear of recurrence often manifests itself as misplaced anger. "The real reason the two of you are fighting is because you're scared and tense that I'll find another cancer," I told the couple. "You need to talk about your feelings, and if you feel like getting angry, direct it at me, not each other."

After cancer, it's sometimes hard for family members to let down their guard. They may feel it's safer to stay pessimistic about the future than risk the potential disappointment of hope. To protect themselves, they end up hiding their fears behind a wall of silence or denial. One patient's son found his mother's breast cancer so upsetting that he failed to call or visit her for months after treatment. Another woman complained that after her chemotherapy for ovarian cancer ended, her sister stopped coming to see her. "She told me she was afraid she'd start crying when she saw I had no hair," says Molly, sixty-eight. "But what I really needed was for us to sit and cry together. Her staying away only hurt me more and made me feel that she'd never love me or share her feelings with me again."

There also are times when a survivor or her family may bury their concerns beneath a mantle of false optimism and vitality. Though it's natural to want to get on with life after cancer and enjoy all that the well world has to offer, some women end up overworking and overcommitting themselves as a way of masking their true fears and feelings. "While Gillian was having chemotherapy, I'd dream of the day she'd be well and we could do things together again," remembers her husband, Jonathan. "Now that treatment is over, she's back to working until eight, nine, ten o'clock at night. I'm proud of her for jumping back to life so quickly. But I'm also worried if she doesn't slow down, she'll end up getting sick again."

Fear of losing your loved one is a common concern for many family members after cancer. Even today, a full two years since my treatments ended, my husband gets depressed if I raise the subject of my cancer coming back. Just the other evening, when the two of us were discussing where we'd like to retire, I said jokingly, "Well, if my cancer returns, at least I'll be in a beautiful place when I die." With that he headed straight to the bedroom and buried himself in a book. To Sheldon there is nothing funny about cancer. A year of suffering through my treatments was enough, and the mere mention of my getting ill again is too painful for him to contemplate.

No one enjoys talking about serious illness and the possibility of death. Cancer is a horribly depressing subject, especially when you're the family member who's lived with it for month upon month. Often a spouse, a parent, or a close friend will avoid discussing the topic, not because they love you any less, but because not talking seems safer and less threatening. Also, after giving such intensive support during treatment, family members often feel so emotionally drained that they want only to put the disease behind them.

Nonetheless, it's important for survivors and their family members to acknowledge what each has been through and to find ways to express their feelings. No matter how long a couple has lived together or how much they have shared in the past, it's impossible to unravel their emotions unless they are brought into the open and spoken aloud.

After operating recently on a sixty-seven-year-old woman for ovarian cancer, I invited her to bring her family to my office to discuss her prognosis. During the meeting, tears welled up in my patient's eyes. "Ever since the second-look operation I've been terrified that my cancer would recur," said Margaret, a retired nurse. "But I haven't told anyone about these fears because I didn't want them to be frightened, too."

Margaret's daughter, who was sitting next to her, leaned over and began crying herself. "Mom, I love you so much," she said. "I knew you were scared and I've been scared, too. But I never said anything because I didn't want you to have to worry about me, too."

There—it was out. They all were frightened, and now this was in the open, I could see a measure of relief spread across their faces. It didn't make sense to hide anymore from what they were feeling. Like a release of the floodgates, all the family began to cry and tell each other how terrifying the experience had been.

Opening Up

Sharing feelings and fears can be important emotional medicine. But it also can be terribly painful. As a survivor, you may need to take that first frightening step, showing your family you are ready and willing to open up and discuss how cancer has affected you. It's probably unrealistic to expect the other members of your family to volunteer their feelings in some intense outpouring of emotion, but there are more subtle ways to crack open the door to communication.

A survivor might say to her husband or a grown child, "My cancer makes me feel like we've grown apart. Instead of going through our private hells separately, why don't we try sharing some of our feelings together?" A family member also might try telling a survivor: "I know your cancer is hard for both of us to discuss, but if you ever want to talk with me about it, I'm always there to listen." If she doesn't feel like talking about it, she'll tell you; but when you offer, it lets her know that you're not too frightened to hear her feelings.

Having a sounding board can help the survivor focus her anger or anxiety and help her get a clearer sense of where she stands with her feelings about her health, her role in the family, her concerns about finances, or her worries about getting back to work. It also can help a family member feel more involved and needed. On my suggestion, one of my patients with uterine cancer now sets aside an hour each evening to take a stroll with her husband.

"The first few times we danced around the issues, talking about our kids and not ourselves," admits Lorna, fifty-six. "But one evening I told Bill how scared I was about getting the cancer again, and we started to really talk. Now we look forward to having that special time together as a way of keeping our lives connected."

As survivors, each of us will surely experience other hurdles in life. We may need to care for an elderly parent, an ill spouse, a troubled child, or another disease ourselves. There's no telling what the future will bring. But if we learn to keep up an honest dialogue with our loved ones, the emotional health and well-being of our family will surely profit.

Still, some survivors may go through the cancer experience without family members to rely on. As single women, they will need to look for strength and support from their friends. It may be difficult to ask for help, and you may not find solace from one friend alone. Indeed, you may find it uncomfortable to be with some of your friends after cancer and find others who offer more help than you expected. But over time, as you learn to open up and reach out with your emotions, certain relationships will deepen and grow, allowing you to forge your own family of sorts among a few of your closest friends.

For the Children's Sake

Children often have a difficult time adjusting when a survivor comes home after treatment. It's hard for them to know how to cope, especially if their mother or grandmother comes home looking and acting sicker than when she left. They need reassurance that their loved one is back and ready to take care of them. But at first a survivor may feel too drained to take care of anyone other than herself. As a result, children may start acting out their fears and worries, finding it hard to concentrate at school or get along with other kids. They may be more reckless when they play, or they may worry obsessively about getting sick themselves. Their grades may drop or get even better as they throw themselves into their work as an escape.

Any of these changes can occur when a child feels scared or worried, and the best a mother can do is encourage her children to share their feelings, no matter how painful or hurtful they may be.

"My teenage daughter and I have always been close, but when I came home from surgery, she barely said a word to me," says Rita, a thirty-nine-year-old survivor of cervical cancer. "When I asked what was wrong, she mumbled something and sulked off to her room. Finally, one night I sat down at her desk and wrote her a letter about how sad I felt. The next day I found a note on my pillow that read, 'Mom, I really love you, but if I say it out loud, I might lose you.'"

When cancer strikes a parent or a grandparent, some children resent the loss of attention. Others fear their parent may die and leave them alone in the world. When a survivor returns home, a child may find it difficult to resolve their feelings and suddenly begin loving their parent as before. Try to keep communication open with your children and explain to them in simple terms how you're feeling. Like you, they may feel confused and a bit uncertain, and it can help if you express your thoughts first.

In addition, a child may feel upset when she can't share activities with her mother as she did before. When this happens, it can help to look for some activity the entire family can do together and enjoy. "Now that I have nerve pain, I'm afraid to cook," says Connie, whose chemotherapy for ovarian cancer left her with peripheral neuropathy in her hands and feet. "Fortunately, my children have always been great at helping me in the kitchen. After school they help me get out all the ingredients and measure them out. I supervise and they do the actual cooking, so I feel like I'm taking care of them, and they have fun helping me in a way I can't do myself."

It also may help if a favorite relative or family friend can devote some extra time and attention to the children. They may want to take them out for a special outing or help them after school with their homework. Some children find it easier to open up to a grown-up who isn't an authority figure in the family. If these efforts to provide solace and support fail, professional counseling for a child, or child and parent together, may be necessary and shouldn't be overlooked.

Reassuring Your Child about Cancer

Talking about cancer with young children can be difficult, but you need to tell them several important things:

- Having cancer doesn't necessarily mean a person will die from it.
- Nothing you did or didn't do caused Mommy to get cancer.
- Nothing you thought or said caused the cancer to grow.
- Cancer isn't contagious—you can't catch it from someone else.
- Because your mom or grandmother had cancer doesn't always mean you or someone else in your family will get it, too.
- The way you behave can't change the fact that your mom had cancer or that your family is upset.
- It's important to continue with school and outside activities.
- There are others to talk to besides your parents about your fears.

Getting Help

When someone in your family has had cancer, every member is likely to get "sick" as well. Aspirations and plans of the spouse and children, as well as of the survivor herself, must often be readjusted, and roles within the family structure must be redefined. Families who are used to talking openly with each other may be able to work out many of their difficulties together. But larger problems may arise that only professional counseling can help.

To survive ovarian cancer, Eliza was forced to undergo two abdominal surgeries and twelve months of chemotherapy. When her treatments finally ended, the numbness in her hands and feet was so severe that she could barely walk or hold a cane. Terrified to see his wife so debilitated, Eliza's husband immediately rented a wheelchair and hired a nurse's aide to be with her constantly. Every time Eliza attempted to walk, the aide would be at her side. As the weeks passed, Eliza grew sad and despondent.

"I feel like a wilted flower that's only given a drop of water to drink each day," she told me at our first follow-up exam together. "I know that Arthur is trying to protect me, but how will I ever get back my own life, if I'm never allowed to try?"

Eventually, on my recommendation, Eliza sought the help of a psychotherapist who helped her accept her limitations and regain her sense of self-confidence. Over time she was able to express her needs to her husband and to tell him gently but firmly, "I have to do it alone. If I stumble and fall, let me. At least allow me to try."

Often, a loved one's desire to "do something" can end up inadvertently taking away the survivor's sense of control and self-esteem. No one who has had cancer—or any life-threatening illness, for that matter—wants to be made to feel helpless. Yet in their efforts to help, many family members end up placing the survivor in a position of dependency. Cancer attacks one's self-concept as a whole person as well as threatening one's life. Instead of compounding the feelings of helplessness by treating a survivor as an invalid, it's far better to let her pull her own weight and fail, giving her a steady stream of encouragement to keep on trying.

Short-term counseling can help family members recognize these problems and find better and more appropriate ways of expressing their concern. It won't make the feelings hurt any less. Nothing really can. But often it can help survivors and their family members uncover their true fears and uncertainties about cancer and give them strategies to cope.

Role Changes

After cancer, a survivor may have every good intention of plunging right back into life. But after an ordeal as grueling as cancer treatment, this can take some time. At first you may feel a bit overwhelmed to come home and take on your previous role as head of the household. Depending on your level of fatigue or other side effects left over from therapy, you might not be able to handle at first the concurrent roles of wife and mother, disciplinarian and homemaker, wage earner, mediator, and friend.

"I'd always been the parent who threatened to turn off the TV, who set the limits on how late our kids were allowed to stay out, or who doled out punishment when rules were broken," says Lisa, a forty-two-year-old breast cancer survivor. "When I ended treatment I just didn't have the energy, and things around the house started to disintegrate. All the usual patterns disappeared, and our roles seemed to get reversed. Suddenly I became the most dependent member in the family."

Keeping a household together and in sync takes a lot of effort and cooperation. For the health of the entire family, each member must rally together and share the load so the survivor has time to rest and recuperate. This means sitting down together and deciding what routines around the house are important and which can be relaxed for a time. Perhaps you won't have the cleanest house on the block or a gourmet meal every night. And you may have to ask your spouse and friends for help with the shopping or getting the kids to school on time. But there's no shame in shifting responsibilities, especially if it will give you necessary time to recover from the physical and emotional wounds of cancer.

"When my support group heard I'd come home from the hospital, they volunteered to do my cooking for several weeks," says Gladys, sixty-three. "At first I felt a bit uncomfortable accepting their help, but when I look back, I know it's what really enabled me get my strength back."

If outreach is an important part of your church, rotary group, or community center, feel free to ask for help with homemaking tasks or transportation. Ask your children's school if you can sign up with a carpool that will let you fulfill your side of the driving at a later date. There also may be county or private agencies in your area that can provide trained homemakers or licensed home health aides to render some assistance.

Remember, not everything remains the same once you start up your life again, and sometimes it may take a little extra care and attention to get family roles straightened out. The important thing is that you and your loved ones are a family again, and as a family you need to solve problems together. After any serious illness, it can take a bit of time and effort to readjust to day-to-day life and routines, but the key is to keep trying and keep talking—and not be afraid to ask for help.

Nine

FACING MENOPAUSE

*I*t's been three years since I was treated for breast cancer, and knock on wood, I'm still disease-free. But I must confess, I haven't had a decent night's sleep since therapy ended. Every evening I go to bed at ten o'clock, and an hour and a half later, like clockwork, I bolt awake. Out of nowhere a wave of heat hits, drenching me with perspiration from my head to my toes. Kicking off the covers, I slowly drift back to sleep. But an hour later I'm up again, shivering with cold. Two more hours and it's two A.M., when the wave of heat strikes again. Off with my nightgown and back to sleep. Up again an hour later, clammy and chilled. Hot, cold. Asleep. Awake. When women complain miserably about hot flashes, I identify with them completely. The symptoms of menopause are real.

For many cancer survivors, chemotherapy, radiation, or surgery causes a drop in estrogen production that leads to premature menopause. Other survivors may go through the change of life as part of their body's normal aging process. But whatever the cause, the symptoms and consequences of menopause can be disturbing: hot flashes, vaginal dryness, diminished bladder capacity, and insomnia, as well as an increased risk for osteoporosis and heart disease.

For years doctors have routinely prescribed hormone replacement therapy to alleviate or forestall these effects. But the scientific evidence supporting the long-term safety of hormone use still remains poor, with conflicting data. When a woman goes through menopause, she must weight the benefits of taking hormonal therapy against its potential risks. If she also has cancer in her background, the decision becomes even more difficult.

On the one hand, estrogen replacement offers many benefits. It successfully relieves hot flashes and vaginal dryness and prevents osteoporosis, a bone-weakening condition that afflicts 70 percent of women age seventy-five and older. Women taking estrogen replacement also have a lower incidence of heart disease than those who don't. But taking estrogen replacement presents numerous risks for disease, including an increased risk for endometrial cancer and the possible threat of breast cancer as well.

Today, unless a woman has undergone a hysterectomy, doctors routinely add progestin (a synthetic form of progesterone) to hormone replacement therapy to offset estrogen's carcinogenic effects on the uterus. But progestin may counteract estrogen's beneficial effects on the heart and further promote the risk for breast cancer.

For cancer survivors especially, this raises some very troubling questions: If a woman takes hormones to prevent osteoporosis, will she be putting herself at increased risk for breast cancer? If she chooses hormone replacement to alleviate temporary symptoms like hot flashes, is she setting herself up for long-term risks?

Though important ongoing medical studies may eventually provide some answers, they offer little solace to the survivor who is trying to make an informed decision about hormone replacement today. Too often women end up taking hormones because they rely on the erroneous advice of media reports and advertising without having a thorough knowledge of the facts.

Before you make any decisions, you need to go over the scientific evidence with your doctor and balance the benefits of hormone therapy against your own *personal* risks for disease. Depending on the kind of cancer you've had, your lifestyle, and your family's medical history, you still may be able to take hormone therapy. Or there may be alternatives to estrogen and progesterone you might want to try first. But always remember that all drugs, *including hormone replacement*, have a powerful effect on the body, and no woman should embark on any course of therapy until she understands clearly what their short- and long-term consequences could be.

How Hormones Work

The hormones estrogen and progesterone drive the female reproductive cycle. During a woman's childbearing years, her ovaries produce enough of these hormones each month to cause the lining of the uterus to thicken and nourish a fertilized egg; if there is no fertilization, the hormone levels drop, the lining of the uterus breaks down, and menstruation occurs.

These hormones also work in a complex way on other parts of your body. Estrogen raises levels of "good" cholesterol in the blood (HDL) and dilates vessels in the heart that regulate blood flow; estrogen and progesterone also preserve a healthy level of calcium in your bones to keep them strong and resilient.

After age thirty-five the ovaries gradually begin to produce less of these hormones. At about age forty the decline in estrogen production becomes more pronounced and menopause nears. Eventually the ovaries stop producing progesterone but continue to release small amounts of estrogen.

The average age of menopause in the United States is fifty-one, but menopause can begin to occur at any time after age forty and may take as long as five years before monthly periods stop and the body adjusts to the changes in estrogen and progesterone production. However, for one of my patients, Carla, the change was more abrupt. At thirty-nine she was diagnosed with an early breast cancer, mandating lumpectomy with radiation and an eight-month course of chemotherapy. Throughout treatment Carla's one and only thought was survival. But once the ordeal was over, she found it hard to face the fact that chemotherapy had permanently disrupted her body's normal production of estrogen and progesterone.

"I'm already exhausted from the therapy, and now I have to contend with these awful bouts of hot flashes that keep me up most of the night," she complained at a recent follow-up examination. "I'm irritable most of the day, and the one time my husband and I tried to have sex, it was so painful we had to stop."

Like many cancer survivors, Carla was facing the distressing but short-term effects of premature menopause. When cancer forces doctors to remove the ovaries, or give chemotherapy or radiation, the body's normal production of estrogen and progesterone can stop. This shuts down a woman's normal menstrual cycle and may cause symptoms like vaginal dryness, hot flashes, and diminished bladder capacity. Some women also complain that menopause leads to decreased sexual desire, mood swings, irritability, and an inability to concentrate. Even former First Lady Barbara Bush, in her recently published autobiography, attributed her crashing depression in the mid-1970s to the hormonal changes of menopause.

However, the scientific data on mood changes associated with menopause is conflicting. There are many important life changes at the age of menopause. Often it is hard to untangle all the changing variables and attribute any particular one as the sole cause of mood changes. Yet contrary to popular belief, no scientific evidence shows a physiologic link between menopause and depression. Hot flashes are usually worse at night, and the resulting loss of sleep can make a woman irritable and moody during the day. Vaginal dryness often makes sex painful, and anticipating pain can make a woman feel disinterested in sex. But there simply is no medical data that shows menopause directly *causes* these feelings. It may be an association rather than a causation.

Moreover, no studies indicate that hormone replacement can alleviate the emotional problems of middle age, let alone preserve a woman's youthful appearance or prevent wrinkles. Estrogen therapy isn't the miracle therapy it was purported to be when doctors routinely began prescribing it in the 1960s. As I frequently tell my patients, the only symptoms that consistently disappear with hormone replacement are hot flashes and vaginal dryness. The effect of hormone replacement on other symptoms such as irritability, insomnia, and mood swings varies from person to person, depending on the underlying cause of the symptoms and the makeup of the individual.

Even so, when Carla came in that day so distressed, I knew I needed to thoroughly discuss the benefits *and* the risks of hormone replacement with her. Like many women, she'd heard that after the drop in estrogen production during menopause, women begin to lose their natural protection against osteoporosis and heart disease. But I explained that taking hormone replacement therapy to offset these risks may not always be the safest course of action.

Research shows that taking estrogen clearly lessens the risk for bone fractures in older age, but a woman may need to take it for many years, perhaps *forever*, to reap this benefit. A recent study in the *New England Journal of Medicine* suggested that once a woman stops taking hormones, especially if she is under sixty-five, bone loss will be rapid, so that any of the benefits from hormones may be lost. But studies also show that after ten years of estrogen replacement therapy, the risk of breast cancer increases.

What about estrogen therapy's protective effect on the heart? It is true that several recent studies suggest a 50 to 80 percent reduced risk of heart disease and stroke among women who use estrogen. The problem is that much of the research demonstrating the cardiovascular benefits of hormone replacement is based on unopposed estrogen therapy, not the combined estrogen-progesterone regimens in common use today. We don't know the long-term effect of progesterone on heart disease.

The National Institutes of Health has two large studies under way that will compare the effects of estrogen alone versus estrogen with progesterone on heart disease risk, among other things. Early results suggest progesterone does not change the effect of estrogen on HDL (the good cholesterol).

Where does this leave cancer survivors like Carla? Each woman needs to be aware that the benefits of hormone therapy can sometimes be overshadowed by its risks. When you read a health article or drug advertisement that promotes hormone replacement therapy as a way to prevent heart disease and osteoporosis, it may sound as though estrogen and progesterone will be adding years to your life. But in reality, the latest data shows that a woman at risk for breast cancer taking estrogen replacement therapy may actually *shorten* her life span by further increasing her risk for breast and endometrial cancer.

The Cancer Connection

Cancer appears to be a multistep process—in other words, in order for cancer to occur, an individual must be subjected over a lifetime to just the right combination of risk factors. In the case of breast cancer, for example, numerous indicators like age, family history, and incidence of previous cancers can increase a woman's odds for the disease. In addition, research indicates a woman's lifetime exposure to estrogen *and* progesterone may also be a major determinant.

Cancer experts have found that estrogen stimulates cell growth in breast tissue; although progesterone seems to block this proliferative effect of estrogen in the uterus, it has a strangely opposite effect on breast tissue, causing breast cells to replicate over and over again, increasing the chances that a cancerous mutation will occur.

Studies have shown that women who have their ovaries removed early in life, and who are therefore exposed to vastly less estrogen than other women, rarely have breast cancer. Conversely, women who start menstruating early or who go through menopause late have a higher risk for cancer of the breast and uterus. Evidence also shows that women who are overweight after menopause have a higher risk for breast cancer, most likely because body fat itself produces excess levels of estrogen. In addition, recent data indicates that women who took estrogen in the form of DES (diethylstilbestrol) during pregnancy have a moderately increased risk for breast cancer later in life.

As the pool of medical data continues to grow in support of this hormone-risk theory, new concerns have arisen about the safety of taking hormone replacement therapy. Though numerous reports find no relationship between estrogen medication and breast cancer, other studies suggest a clear link between breast cancer and the length of time postmenopausal women take estrogen.

In research carried out by the National Cancer Institute, postmenopausal women who took estrogen for twenty or more years had a 50 percent increased risk of developing breast cancer. In another study, more than twenty-three thousand Swedish women who used replacement hormones (both estrogen and estrogen-progestin combinations) were followed. Initially these women showed only a 10 percent higher incidence of breast cancer than expected. But a more detailed investigation of all the women in the group who developed breast cancer and a random sample of women who did not develop the disease showed that the risk increased to 70 percent above the expected level among women who used the hormone for nine years or more. More recently, doctors found that women who took 0.625 milligrams of a conjugated estrogen like Premarin for fifteen years, beginning at menopause, would have a 66 percent increase in breast cancer risk by age sixty-five.

Based on more recent scientific data, the lifetime probability of developing breast cancer after long-term estrogen use is increased by almost one-third (30 percent). Although this is a modest increase, the disease is already so prevalent that this will clearly have an effect on the total number of women who develop the disease. But still there's a hitch: all studies connecting hormone replacement to breast cancer involve women who took estrogen alone or who took a version of estrogen and progesterone not prescribed in this country. As a consequence, when experts relate this data to women currently on combination therapy, the evidence may or may not be applicable.

Nevertheless, since progesterone has been shown to increase cell division in breast tissue, there is the possibility that combined therapy might also heighten breast cancer risk.

Weighing Your Personal Risks

The safety of hormone replacement regimens—particularly for women with a history of certain cancers—is still extremely controversial. Assessing whether or not to take hormone replacement therapy is no easy task and depends largely on your own risk factors for disease. Too often advertisements in magazines and newspapers make it seem as if hormones should be a universal prescription for every woman. The truth is, there are some cases when a woman definitely should not take hormone therapy and other cases when the benefits outweigh the risks. To decide, you need to carefully evaluate your personal health history, factoring what kind of cancer you had, what kinds of cancer other family members may have had, and what other medical problems you have currently or have had in the past.

In my patient Carla's case, for instance, I strictly advised her *not* to take hormones. Not only had she herself had breast cancer, but her mother developed uterine cancer at age fifty-five, indicating Carla's family might have a genetic tendency for hormonally driven cancers. If she took combined therapy, she might further increase her risk for recurrence or for a secondary cancer in her breast.

Also, until more scientific data is available, I'm wary about prescribing hormone therapy for patients who have had endometrial cancer. Florence, a fifty-five-year-old kindergarten teacher, had been on estrogen replacement therapy for five years because of severe menopausal symptoms of vaginal dryness, sweats, and flushes and a family history of osteoporosis. The hormones had alleviated her symptoms and, presumably, slowed her bone loss. But when she began breakthrough bleeding, her gynecologist advised a uterine biopsy. Results showed cancerous cell changes in her endometrium, and she was referred to me for surgery.

Fortunately the cancer in Florence's uterus was contained, and after performing a total hysterectomy, I deemed further chemotherapy or radiation unnecessary. But when she consulted me about resuming hormone therapy, I cautioned her against it. She didn't have any symptoms to justify further therapy, and even though her uterus had been completely removed and her risk for recurrence essentially eliminated, her cancer placed her in higher danger of developing a second cancer in her breasts. We discussed what is known about the relationship between estrogen and breast cancer and decided the risks of further cancer outweighed its benefits. However, to minimize her potential for osteoporosis, I strongly advised Florence to begin an exercise program and supplement her diet with 1,500 mg of calcium and 400 IU of vitamin D.

For patients like Florence, I also monitor bone loss by obtaining annual bone densitometry. I also monitor their cardiac risk factors and obtain stress tests, EKG, and lipid profiles. If a woman's risk for heart disease or osteoporosis becomes apparent, I may then reassess her need for hormones.

Who Should Not Take Hormone Therapy?

Do cancer survivors who already have a heightened risk for recurrence and second cancers further increase their odds by taking hormone replacement therapy? No one really knows. Because the current hormone replacement regimens have not been around for that long, we still do not have a clear picture regarding long-term risks of hormone use—especially for women who have survived cancer. Still, it needs to be understood that in general, once a woman has had cancer, her risks are significantly increased for developing a second cancer in any part of her body, particularly for certain kinds of cancer like breast, colon, ovarian, and uterine.

Breast cancer and uterine cancer are the two main contraindications for hormone replacement. However, some small studies have shown that a number of women with endometrial cancer can be given hormones. Your doctor will need to review the kind of uterine cancer you had and the risk of hormone replacement.

More data may soon be forthcoming from a national study investigating estrogen use in patients. Known as the PEPI trial, this study will help us understand the short-*and* long-term risks of hormone replacement and which women will most benefit from their use.

Nevertheless, if you have a history of blood clots, you should not take hormone therapy. Studies show that women using high-dose estrogen in birth control pills are at increased risk of developing inflammation of the veins (phlebitis), which can lead to life-threatening blood clots in the lungs (pulmonary embolism). This risk increases if a woman smokes. Research on postmenopausal women taking hormone replacement suggests they may face a similar risk if they have had a history of phlebitis.

Family history for breast cancer is also important to consider when deciding whether or not to institute hormone replacement therapy and/or whether to continue such therapy for many years. Researchers have shown that a woman with a family history of breast cancer—particularly when it appears before menopause in both breasts—has one of the highest risks of getting the disease herself. If you or a family member has had cancer of the ovary, colon, or endometrium, that also raises your risk for getting breast cancer, and taking hormone therapy may up your risks, although the data is controversial.

If you are overweight, you may also need to be cautious about taking hormone replacement. Studies reveal that a high-fat diet and obesity lead to a higher production of estrogen in a woman's body. It stands to reason that if the breasts are already being stimulated by excess estrogen, it may not be wise to stimulate them any further. How hormone replacement affects a woman's breasts for the long term—meaning five to ten years—still isn't known. But I find it alarming that many doctors continue to prescribe hormone therapy indefinitely, particularly when there's been no in-depth look at its long-term consequences. Weight loss, exercise, and dietary counseling, with or without hormone replacement, would be a safer bet.

Women who have had severe liver disease or gallbladder disease are usually advised not to take hormone replacement, either. Bile, which helps in the digestion of food, is produced and stored in the gallbladder. Unless estrogen is given transdermally (by a skin patch), the hormone passes through the liver before entering the bloodstream, where it can thicken and concentrate the bile, increasing the risk of gallstones. These gallstones can cause infection and painful irritation in the gallbladder. They can also obstruct the flow of bile into the intestinal tract. Studies have shown that women using estrogen are two and a half times more likely to get gallbladder disease than women who do not take hormones.

I also advise women with the following conditions to carefully weigh the pros and cons of hormone replacement therapy:

- uterine fibroids: The fibroids may grow on estrogens. If you decide to take them, careful gynecologic follow-up is needed.
- migraine headaches: Estrogens seem to make headaches worse.
- endometriosis: Theoretically this condition can be exacerbated by estrogen.
- past use of DES: Recent studies show that women who took the estrogen derivative DES (diethylstilbestrol) during pregnancy have a 35 to 40 percent greater than normal chance of developing breast cancer. Experts theorize that taking hormone replacement therapy could possibly exacerbate this risk.
- history of melanoma: Research shows that melanoma may be hormonally sensitive. One recent case study described a woman on estrogen therapy who then developed a flare-up of this serious form of skin cancer.

Who Should Take Hormones?

Only you and your physician can decide if—and when—hormone therapy is right for you. I usually advise my patients with hormonally related cancers to try less controversial remedies to alleviate symptoms like hot flashes and vaginal dryness. Other women, however, who have had non-hormone-related cancers (cervical cancer or

Hodgkin's disease, for example) may feel the benefits of taking hormones outweigh their risks.

The National Women's Health Network, a Washington-based research group, recommends the use of hormone therapy only for premenopausal women who have had their ovaries removed prematurely, for women who experience extreme menopausal discomforts, and for women who are at high risk of fractures from osteoporosis. I concur with their recommendations, but for cancer survivors I need to add one proviso. If you've had your ovaries removed because of cancer of the ovary or uterus *or* if there's a strong family history of cancer of the ovary, uterus, breast, or colon, you may be part of a family cancer syndrome that puts you at increased risk for breast cancer. As a consequence, you may decide that taking estrogen, because of its small to moderate increase in risk, is simply not worth the worry.

Moreover, proponents of hormones frequently point to evidence that cardiovascular disease is the number-one killer of women. But the tables of risk appear to be turning. A recent review in the *Journal of the American Medical Association* shows that by the year 2000, cancer, *not* heart disease, will be the leading cause of death in this country. Recently a physician referred a fifty-seven-year-old accountant named Sarah to me for counseling about hormone replacement. She had had a minor skin cancer, but when she arrived for her first visit, her main concern was heart disease. Sarah was massively obese—close to 250 pounds.

"My internist thinks I should be taking estrogen to prevent heart disease," she told me matter-of-factly. "Do you think hormone replacement will help?"

"If you're truly interested in your heart," I answered candidly, "you have to begin losing weight."

For the next half hour I explained how years of overeating and a sedentary lifestyle had placed her not only at risk of heart disease, but also in danger of endometrial, colon, and breast cancer. One little pill of estrogen a day was not going to undo those risks. What she really needed to do was make a concerted effort to lose weight and begin a regular walking program that would probably have greater benefits on her heart than taking hormone replacement alone. A supervised weight loss program centered around behavior modification rather than "binge" dieting would help with *sustained* weight loss.

On the other hand, I've seen cases where the benefit of taking hormone replacement probably outbalances the risks—specifically in women who have a severe risk of osteoporosis. Virginia, a fifty-three-year-old lawyer and fifteen-year survivor of Hodgkin's disease, came to see me recently, wondering if she should be on estrogen therapy. Her eighty-year-old mother had fallen the year before and fractured her hip. Virginia realized that her mother's history of osteoporosis, as well as her own lack of exercise, placed her at high risk as well. But she also was concerned about hormone therapy's connection to cancer.

"Before I can recommend hormone therapy," I told her, "we need to determine how much mineral loss your bones have gone through already."

When her test results came back, bone densitometry scans showed that Virginia had a tendency toward mild osteoporosis. Since there was no history of breast cancer in her family, but her father had died of heart disease, we agreed that the benefits of hormone treatment outweighed its potential risks. By taking a combination therapy of estrogen with progestin, she would reduce the likelihood of endometrial cancer while enhancing her protection against osteoporosis. On my recommendation she also began supplementing her diet with calcium and working out with an exercise trainer three times a week. She would need to get annual mammograms and screen herself monthly for breast lumps. As a final safeguard, I recommended we reassess her need for treatment yearly, but particularly at age sixty-three, by which time she will have been on hormone replacement for ten years.

If you and your physician decide that hormone therapy is warranted to treat specific menopausal symptoms or osteoporosis, make certain your doctor prescribes the lowest dose that is effective for your individual case. Before hormone replacement is begun, a pretreatment mammogram should be taken. It also is especially important that a cancer survivor on hormone replacement therapy be checked several times each year for any signs of new disease. Vaginal bleeding should be reported to your doctor at once. Also, a woman taking estrogen should examine her breasts monthly for lumps or changes in appearance that may be warning signs of cancer, and she should have yearly mammograms to watch for signs of breast disease.

Alternatives to Hormone Therapy

If you are not a candidate for hormone therapy—or the idea of taking hormones just doesn't feel right to you—alternative treatments for menopausal problems are available. Survivors of breast cancer, endometrial cancer, and other medical conditions that preclude hormone replacement may still have risk factors for osteoporosis and cardiovascular disease; they also may suffer from severe menopausal symptoms that require treatment. Certain nonhormonal medications are effective in reducing hot flashes and related symptoms, and other changes in lifestyle can help prevent osteoporosis and heart disease. Before you make any decisions, talk with your physician about your medical needs and risk factors to see which combination of remedies may work best for you.

Vaginal Dryness

As a woman's estrogen production dwindles, her vagina may become drier and less elastic, a condition called vaginal atrophy. This change may create some difficulty and discomfort with sexual intercourse, but there are remedies that help. Several over-the-counter vaginal lubricants can replenish a woman's natural secretions, but some experimentation may be required before she finds one that works best for her (see page 104).

To make sex more comfortable, it is also important to have intercourse or use a vaginal dilator at least two to three times per week.

Regular stretching of the vaginal wall will make intercourse less painful. If you have intercourse less than once or twice a week, ask your physician for a dilator so that when you do have sex, the vagina will have maintained its patency and will be less painful.

Hot Flashes

Hot flashes are among the most common—and troublesome—symptoms of menopause. Sudden waves of heat in the upper part of the body are usually accompanied by a rising flushing of the chest, neck, and face and are often followed by heavy sweating, dizziness, heart palpitations, and headache. Soon after, a woman may experience a cold, clammy feeling as her body tries to readjust.

Each episode can last from a few seconds to a few minutes, but in severe cases a hot flash may endure for five minutes or more. While these heat waves are more likely to occur at night, they can be disruptive whenever they happen, whether at a business meeting, a social gathering, or in the midst of a deep sleep.

Though their cause is not clearly understood, hot flashes most likely are triggered when the drop in estrogen stimulates the hypothalamus, a gland in the brain that regulates body temperature. Over time, as a woman's body learns to adjust to lesser amounts of estrogen, hot flashes begin to diminish and eventually disappear. However, women on tamoxifen may continue to have hot flashes as long as they are on the medication.

Even though hormone replacement is perhaps the most immediate way to relieve the discomfort of hot flashes, there are other medications a woman might try first. Megestrol acetate (Megace), a progesterone-like drug used primarily for treating advanced cancers of the breast and uterus, has been useful in stemming hot flashes. However, its long-term side effects are uncertain, and women with liver disease or a history of blood clots are advised against taking the drug. Megace also may increase the risk of breast cancer.

In addition, two blood pressure medications, alpha-methyldopa (Aldomet) and clonidine hydrochloride (Catapres), seem to be helpful against hot flashes. However, women with active liver disease are advised to avoid methyldopa.

In lieu of taking medication to curb hot flashes, many women find physical exercise helpful. During exercise the brain releases chemicals known as endorphins, which are thought to alleviate the flushes. In a recent study, physically active postmenopausal women were much less likely to suffer from moderate and severe hot flashes than their sedentary counterparts. There is also evidence that caffeine and alcohol can exacerbate hot flashes. Avoiding coffee, tea, colas, and chocolate, as well as limiting alcoholic beverages, may help control your symptoms.

Osteoporosis Prevention

In women who cannot take hormone replacement therapy, exercise is particularly crucial for preventing osteoporosis. Recent studies show that women who engage in active fitness programs that include weight-bearing exercises have higher bone densities than sedentary women. Weight-bearing exercises include low-impact aerobics, resistance training, jogging, power walking, and other activities that involve the use of large muscles to resist counterpressure; in contrast, swimming and casual walking cause only minimal changes in bone density. Stress placed on the bone by muscles during exercise is thought to cause an increase in the activity of bone-forming cells, which results in a buildup of bone density.

Even if a woman is unaccustomed to exercising, she can increase her bone density with a moderate program of fast walking alternated with ten to fifteen repetitions a day of low-weight lifting. I'm not talking about some sort of Sly Stallone–type workout here—just a regular and consistent program that involves walking briskly for a half hour three times a week and lifting two- to three-pound arm and leg weights every other day.

In addition, all women need to consume 1,500 milligrams of calcium daily to maintain an adequate mineral balance in their bones. This can be taken in supplement form and by regular consumption of calcium-rich foods like dairy products, broccoli, soybeans, and green leafy vegetables such as spinach and kale. Keep in mind, too, that smoking, as well as excess use of caffeine and alcohol, can increase the loss of calcium through your stool and urine. Also, long-term use of thyroid or cortisone-like medication can leach calcium from your bones or prevent adequate calcium absorption.

Though it's impossible to determine from your appearance whether you're truly at risk for osteoporosis, women who have a small, thin frame or who are Caucasian or Asian seem to have a higher risk for the disease. Family history is another strong risk factor. In the same way that women have annual mammograms, doctors are moving toward annual preventative screening for osteoporosis. New and better methods of measuring bone density can help predict how likely you are to develop this bone-brittling disease. Most major medical centers now have bone densitometry (DEXA) machines to precisely gauge the weight and density of a woman's bones. Your doctor may prescribe a baseline measurement to evaluate where you stand at the beginning of menopause. She'll then be able to compare it to tests taken annually to evaluate whether your regimen of exercise and diet is alone enough to prevent bone loss from aging.

If your doctor finds your bones are beginning to lose their density, the nonhormonal drug calcitonin can help forestall further symptoms. Several studies have demonstrated that calcitonin produces a beneficial effect on bone metabolism and bone density within one to three years of initiating treatment. Unfortunately calcitonin is expensive and must be administered through the nose to be most effective. In several years, however, you may be a candidate for a new class of drugs under investigation called biphosphanates, which already have shown great promise for the treatment of osteoporosis.

What about Tamoxifen?

Another alternative to estrogen therapy that is showing encouraging, even lifesaving benefits is the synthetic hormonelike drug tamoxifen.

Known to block the proliferative effect of estrogen in the breast, tamoxifen has been used for close to twenty years to treat patients with advanced breast cancer. Since 1985 it also has been recommended in the United States for "adjuvant," or additional, therapy following radiation and lumpectomy for early stage breast cancer. The drug is also being studied in the United States and abroad as a chemopreventative—in other words, a method to prevent breast cancer.

Today tamoxifen is one of the most widely prescribed drugs in the world. Thousands of breast cancer survivors are currently taking the drug not only to prevent recurrence, but also to forestall the development of new cancers in the opposite breast. Studies also suggest that tamoxifen may be just as effective as estrogen replacement therapy to reduce blood cholesterol levels and help maintain bone density in postmenopausal women.

Though tamoxifen has shown limited side effects in patients with breast cancer, it does tend to cause hot flashes, vaginal discharge, and irregular bleeding in approximately a quarter of women who use it. Like estrogen, tamoxifen is also associated with an increased risk of thromboembolic (clotting) disease. In addition, numerous studies indicate a two- to threefold risk of endometrial cancer in women receiving tamoxifen therapy.

So how does a woman decide whether tamoxifen is right for her? If she's had breast cancer, chances are her doctor has already suggested she take the drug to prevent recurrence or a second cancer in her remaining breast. Like many breast cancer survivors, I take my daily dose of tamoxifen each morning, confident that it's raising my chances for a long and healthy life. Sure, I may have to deal with those troublesome bouts of hot flashes and get myself checked by a gynecologist twice a year for endometrial cancer, but that's a lot less worrisome than the fear of grappling with a recurrence or second case of breast cancer.

In the next few years, when more scientific data is available, survivors of other cancers may also be eligible for tamoxifen as a preventative treatment for breast cancer. A large-scale study of the drug is now under way at the National Cancer Institute. The National Breast Cancer Prevention Trial, which includes sixteen thousand women at risk for developing breast cancer, is currently investigating tamoxifen's cardiovascular benefits, its effect on the endometrium and on bones, and its usefulness in preventing breast cancer, along with any harmful side effects it may cause. Due for completion in the late 1990s, this trial should enable doctors and patients to better define the role of tamoxifen in the treatment of menopause.

Until then, it is incumbent on all cancer survivors to thoroughly discuss the management of menopause with their oncologist. Each woman's medical history is different, and only your doctor can help you evaluate which specific risks and benefits you face by taking hormonal therapy or an alternative form of treatment. No doubt the advertisements you read for estrogen and progesterone medication may sound convincing, and your friends or family members may have positive experiences to share. But you're the one who has survived cancer, and you owe it to yourself to take the safest course possible not only to lessen the symptoms of menopause, but also to live the longest and healthiest life possible.

Ten

STRESS, LONELINESS, AND DEPRESSION

*T*he alarm went off at seven A.M., but Coreen had been awake for hours. There were unpaid medical bills to worry about and her upcoming appointment at the oncologist's. Last night's dinner dishes lay piled in the kitchen sink, the laundry needed folding, and if she hurried, she could still get to the market before her nine-thirty meeting with clients. But when she reached to turn off the clock radio, Coreen's arm knocked against her favorite perfume bottle, sending it crashing to the floor.

"Suddenly I was crying like a little child," remembers the forty-eight-year-old breast cancer survivor. "Here I'd spent a year of my life struggling to recover, and now all the responsibilities—the house, the job, the bills—seemed so overwhelming. I just felt like crawling under the covers to hide."

After cancer, every woman experiences days when her patience and emotions are tried to the limit. Often survivors must face the continuing demands of work, of raising children, and of keeping house, while balancing concerns about their health and the possibility of recurrent illness. Others may fight off feelings of isolation and depression as they cope with a battered self-image, altered relationships, or circumstances that force them to face recovery alone.

Though we all lead different lives, each of us has days when our confidence fails and the uncertainty of our future overwhelms us. To cope, many women use different techniques—meditation, relaxation tapes, visual imagery exercises, or physical activity—to help them relax and manage their feelings. Some of my patients have told me that attending support groups, talking regularly with their pastor or rabbi, or listening to comforting music takes the edge off their negative emotions. There are even times when venting bad feelings with a good, long cry seems to help.

But should the stress build up and your sadness or loneliness become chronic, it may be time to seek outside counseling or professional therapy. Otherwise it could have an unwanted effect on the good health and well-being you've struggled so hard to achieve.

The Body/Mind Connection

Although there still is no proven link between cancer and the emotions, some investigators have found an associated risk between stress-related anxiety and a lowered immunity to disease. Ongoing studies have shown that when the body is subjected to prolonged stress, a stream of hormones is released into the bloodstream, inhibiting or suppressing the immune system. It is theorized that when the immune system is impaired for an extended period, cancer-promoting substances—like hormones, nicotine, or perhaps even a virus—may move in and travel through the body, coupling with a weak genetic link in the uterus, the breast, the colon, or some other susceptible organ. These multiple factors may incite cancer cells to mutate and a malignant tumor or recurrence to grow. Normally the body would be able to stave off these microscopic beginnings of cancer, but because of a lowered immunity, they may have a chance to dig their trench a bit deeper.

Conversely, other studies indicate that a positive attitude may actually help survivors bolster their body's ability to fend off disease. One cancer research team studied sixty-nine women who had breast cancer, classifying their responses to illness: those who were feistier, who showed a fighting spirit, were twice as likely to survive five years than those who were into stoic acceptance or who felt hopeless about their future. Another study linked passive personality with faster progression of malignant melanoma, a serious skin cancer. More recently an investigation by Stanford researchers found that women with metastatic breast cancer who joined support groups lived twice as long as those without such networks.

Still, a great deal of controversy surrounds the purported connection between the emotions and illness, and more research needs to be done before doctors have a clear understanding of the relationship, if there is any at all. As an oncologist, I know that attitudes and feelings can be positive, life-enhancing forces in a woman's ongoing battle to survive cancer. But this is not to say that emotions "cause" cancer or that bad thoughts or feelings are responsible for a person's failure to recover from disease. Though a good mental outlook is very important, it can't overcome the "biology" of a particularly virulent tumor. Therefore women shouldn't be made to feel guilty if they feel lousy or vulnerable about having had cancer.

However, I'm convinced that the more women make an effort to cope with the negative feelings in their lives, the more they'll be giving themselves *the chance* to enjoy life and keep cancer at bay. Likewise, if limiting the stress in our lives has even a remote possibility of helping us to stay survivors, we might as well give it a shot.

Limiting Stress

Several months ago a patient named Rose came to visit me for a routine follow-up after ovarian cancer. Though she was nearly three years into remission, I could see that she was very upset.

"My son is getting married," she said, almost breaking down in tears.

I remembered her telling me the year before how worried she was about him still being a bachelor at thirty-five, so I told her what great news this seemed to be.

"No, the woman is pregnant," she muttered, wringing her hands.

"But that's wonderful, you'll be a grandmother," I countered.

"In my generation, we don't see it that way," said Rose. "It's an embarrassment, a shame."

"But in this day and age," I said, trying to comfort her, "it doesn't have to be viewed that way. Instead you should go on with your life and look forward to the marriage, to the birth of the child."

Then, suddenly, she looked me straight in the eye and said, "You know, Dr. Runowicz, you're right. I'm not going to give myself cancer again by worrying about it. When I got sick the first time, my brother was going through a divorce. That stress made my cancer grow, and if I don't watch out, all the worry I've been feeling will make my cancer come back."

As a doctor and a scientist, I know Rose's cancer had probably started years before any particularly stressful moment in her life. But I had to give her credit: she'd decided to make an effort not to worry, perhaps giving herself a better chance at survival. The problem is, unless most of us quit our jobs or languish at a health spa every day, it's impossible to eliminate completely the anxiety and tension from our lives. Instead we have to learn how to live with stress and develop successful coping strategies to get us through the day-to-day pressures. To help, here are a few techniques many of my patients and friends have found useful.

- *Start moving.* Like many women, I use exercise to cut my stress. A brisk walk for an hour on Saturday and Sunday puts me in a more relaxed mood and gives me a chance to think things over in low-anxiety surroundings. It frees me from constantly ringing phones, from conversation, and from responsibility; it also gets my endorphins pumping so that when I get back, I'm refreshed and full of energy. Another of my patients tries to play a set or two of tennis at the end of every day; if it's raining or too cold, she hops on her treadmill for a half hour before bed. "If I don't exercise, it's like pressing on the accelerator and the brake at the same time," she says. "Exercise takes the brake off, letting my body reduce its stress naturally."

• *Get in touch with nature.* On most days, especially in winter, few of us have a chance to get outside and breathe the fresh air. We're stuck at a desk or inside our homes. Taking a break to look out at the water or dig in our gardens can refresh the mind and allow us to focus on the present, giving us a moment's escape from the ever-growing list of things to do.

• *Water therapy.* As simple as it sounds, a long, hot shower or a generous soak in the tub is one of the best ways to relieve stress and ease any associated muscle strain. Spritz some favorite perfume in the air, light a candle, and stretch yourself out in the warm water, taking deep breaths and repeating the word *calm* to yourself. After fifteen minutes you'll be amazed at how much more relaxed you feel.

• *Yoga as meditation.* Rena, a New York City accountant and ten-year survivor of breast cancer, has been practicing yoga since the day she ended treatment. After work each night, she lies on her back in a quiet room, her legs outstretched, arms at her sides, and her palms facing up. "I close my eyes and feel my spine 'melt' into the floor," she explains. "Then, starting with my feet and working my way up, I mentally instruct each part of my body to relax. In ten minutes I'm much more refreshed and ready to deal with getting dinner on the table and the rest of the household chores."

• *Consider new work.* A job that challenges your skills and intelligence can lead to greater happiness, but work that's too time-consuming or difficult may promote anxiety and stress. New research reveals that suffering job-related stress—ranging from tension with a boss to getting fired—may raise your risk for colorectal cancer. In a study of more than one thousand adults, doctors from California and Sweden found that those who experienced job stress over the last ten years were five times more likely to develop colorectal cancer than those who did not.

• *Eat right.* Besides lowering the body's immune system and suppressing its tumor-fighting ability, stress may also cause people to engage in chronically unhealthy eating habits, say researchers. Additionally, a poor diet can cause a drop in blood sugar levels, making a person feel tense and irritable because it triggers the release of stress hormones. To keep your stress levels low, cut out the junk food and eat a low-fat, high-fiber diet.

• *Stay away from alcohol*. Relaxing occasionally with a glass of wine doesn't hurt, but using alcohol to mask painful feelings can be dangerous. After its effects wear off, alcohol produces rebound irritability; it also has been linked to an increased risk for cancer of the breast.

• *Look for the lighter side*. For a recent business trip, one of my patients brought along *The 2,000-Year-Old Man* by Mel Brooks and Carl Reiner. "It's such an uproariously funny book," she says, "that when I read a couple of pages between client meetings, it helped me to stay in a good mood and eased a lot of the stress that normally would have built up."

• *Visual imagery*. This autohypnosis technique can help relieve stress before your next appointment at the doctor's or anytime you're feeling on edge and nervous. Go someplace private—to your bedroom, a ladies' room at work, or a peaceful outdoor spot—where you won't be disturbed. Close your eyes, breathe deeply, and try to imagine, as vividly as you can, a place where you feel safe and comfortable. It might be a memory from your childhood, a resort where you vacationed, or an imaginary land. Hold the image—complete with sounds and scents—in your mind for a few minutes. With practice you'll learn to do this exercise quickly and use it to ease stress in almost any situation.

• *Plan ahead*. Research shows that early morning is the time of day many women feel the most tension and anxiety. Often they're racing to work, feeding the kids, and negotiating schedules when their threshold for stress may be lowest. To avoid chaos, stress experts suggest advanced planning—lay out clothes the night before, ask your husband to feed the kids, and set up chores and activities before the morning's last minute scramble hits.

• *Take control*. Worrying is a natural part of life, but it's important to distinguish which concerns are within your control and which are not. For instance, instead of fretting about recurrence, you need to take a proactive approach: screen yourself for disease, see your physician regularly, eat right, and get plenty of exercise. Also, educate yourself about recurrences and second cancers, and heed early warning signs. Beyond that, there's nothing else you can do.

- *Don't sweat the small stuff.* When one of my patients felt pulled in a million different directions, she took out a file card and wrote down six things that were really important in her life, then referred to the card several times each day. "Now, instead of worrying about everything, I have six top-priority items," says Marla, a former ovarian cancer patient. "It's helped me see that talking to my son at bedtime is a whole lot more important than doing the dishes."
- *Group support.* After cancer, many women complain they feel separate and different from the rest of the well world. When you talk over feelings with survivors like yourself, it can help ease the burden of isolation and enable you to find strategies for dealing with fears of recurrence, mending family relationships, and fending off worries about other health concerns.
- *Music clears the mind.* Studies show that playing or listening to music can slow breathing and heart rate, helping you become—and stay—calm. If you're feeling edgy, try listening to a favorite CD or tape. Music is one of the most powerful tools we have to collect the emotions and bring tranquillity to a harried day.
- *Seize the day.* Most survivors agree that after cancer, they have a new appreciation of life. To keep that feeling active and alive, one of my patients tacked a note on her refrigerator that read "Live today as if it were your last." "When I look at it, I'm reminded of how much I've gone through to be a survivor," says Hilary, fifty-seven, five years free of uterine cancer. "Now, when I feel angry or resentful toward someone, I think of my affirmation, and it defuses the tension."

Fighting Loneliness

After cancer, many survivors have to cope with the powerful and painful emotions of loneliness. They may feel isolated and misunderstood, disconnected and separate from their friends, their family, and the world. They also may have to cope with the struggles of life all by themselves, without love, without guidance, and without support.

"My husband died from a heart attack three years ago, and I just finished treatment for breast cancer," says Leona, a sixty-nine-year-old homemaker. "I want to talk with my friends about all these frightening feelings I've been having, but it seems to make them uncomfortable. More and more I find myself alone, crying through much of the day."

One of the saddest aspects of surviving cancer is learning to deal with lost or altered friendships. Though some friends will deal well with your illness and continue to provide support after treatment, others may be unable to cope with the possibility of your death and withdraw from your life. There also will be times when certain friends may try to help but feel uncomfortable or unsure how to go about it. This can make you feel painfully alone and isolated, largely because you're left to fend by yourself with concerns about recurrence and the uncertainty of your own future.

"I have a very devoted and loving husband, and children who truly care," says Lillian, a fifty-nine-year-old colon cancer survivor. "But during the day, when they're all busy at work, I have the sense that I'm being deserted. I don't have the energy to do the things I used to do with my friends or go to the places we used to go. So I end up feeling awful about myself and the life I've been forced to lead."

People express their loneliness in a range of different ways. Like Leona, some women find themselves withdrawn and depressed, unable to communicate their feelings to others. Others, like Lillian, may become self-critical or self-absorbed, irritable or upset. Coping with the aftermath of cancer can wear down the best of us, and each survivor needs to give herself permission to feel lousy and blue—at least for a time.

After a while, however, if loneliness persists, it can lead to a more chronic and unhealthy state of depression, preventing you from reaching out to others. So before that happens, you need to take steps to involve yourself in different activities and choose constructive ways to fill your time. If you are not working outside the home, here are a few techniques to try:

- *Keep learning.* Take a class or try a new sport or hobby that interests you and involves you with other people. Check the bulletin board at the library or get a schedule of continuing education classes from your local high school or college.
- *Volunteer.* Nearby hospitals and day care centers always need a helping hand. Doing something you enjoy that benefits others can be a wonderful buffer against loneliness, allowing you to meet new friends and develop an emotional support network. Your doctor would probably welcome your involvement in talking to new patients or visiting patients in the hospital and serving as a positive role model. I remember how, the morning after my own surgery, I lay in a hospital bed, thinking I'd never be normal again. As I started to feel sorry for myself, in walked my friend Jane, a three-year survivor of breast cancer who had just finished running the New York City marathon at age fifty-seven. Her upbeat attitude really cheered me up and gave me hope that in time I too would be better than ever.
- *Share your talents.* Offer to tutor neighborhood children, teach in an adult literacy program, or use your skills for a local political or environmental cause. You also may want to offer to baby-sit for a friend. Months after one of my patients had recovered from surgery and radiation for cervical cancer, I noticed she was gloomy and putting on weight. When I recommended she get a job or work as a volunteer, she looked at me as though I were from another planet. "Keeping house is the only job I've ever had," she explained. "What possible job could I get at the age of fifty-nine?" When I suggested she volunteer for a local youth group or after-school program, she seemed disinterested. But when I saw her six months later, her weight was down by seven pounds and she looked terrific. "I started baby-sitting for my next-door neighbor," she said, proudly displaying a snapshot of the three-year-old little girl. "She's a real corker—keeps me busy all the time and tires me out—but it's sort of like having a granddaughter of my very own."

- *Welcome new people.* Deliver a meal you've prepared, or offer to show a new couple around your area. It will get you out of the house and make you feel supportive and involved.
- *Reach out on the phone.* If you're unable to leave the house, your local community center, religious affiliation, or cancer support group may have phone outreach programs you can use. Check the local listings in your phone book or ask your doctor for advice.
- *Write a letter.* Jot down your feelings in a note to a friend or send a funny bedtime story to a grandchild who's far away. When you post something in the mail, most often you'll get a return note in several weeks' time.

Treating Depression

Most cancer survivors experience some sadness following treatment as they reflect on what they've been through and what lies ahead for them in life. They may question their altered appearance, their ability to cope with the physical consequences of therapy, their sexual identity, and any adjustments they must make in career and family goals. Added to these worries is the ever-present threat of recurrence that stalks, to varying degrees, every woman who has had cancer. It's only normal to go through a grieving period where you mourn the losses of your past life and worry about what the future has in store. But, over time, if this mourning process doesn't resolve itself and give way to more hopeful thoughts and aspirations, you may be suffering from major depression and need the help of a trained psychotherapist or psychiatrist.

After cancer, common signs of major depression can include:

- persistent sad or "empty" mood
- loss of interest or pleasure in ordinary activities, including sex
- prolonged fatigue or lack of energy
- sleep disturbances, including insomnia, early morning waking, or oversleeping

- loss of appetite and weight, or weight gain
- difficulty concentrating, remembering, making decisions
- feelings of guilt, worthlessness, hopelessness
- suicidal thoughts
- excessive crying
- alcohol or drug abuse, including prescription medications

If you're experiencing any of the above symptoms, talk to your doctor. Suffering from depression isn't something to be ashamed of and can often be alleviated with short-term counseling or medication. If your doctor decides you need outside help, she may refer you to a psychotherapist or psychiatrist with whom you can talk through the experience of your illness and work out feelings of despair and sadness. There will be no "brainwashing," and you will not be told you *must* do anything. Nor does it mean you are weak or "going crazy." Depression following a life-threatening illness like cancer is not the fault of the survivor and may develop for medical—as well as psychological—reasons.

When I discovered what a difficult time my patient Lillian was having coping with her loneliness, I referred her to a psychiatrist on my staff who is specially skilled to deal with the stress and depression following cancer therapy. With the help of antidepressant medication and several months of counseling, Lillian now feels more hopeful about life. "I was trying to do it all on my own," she says. "But I've learned that sometimes you have to reach out for help to get your life back on track."

Staying Happy

Just recently a patient of mine named Connie was readmitted to the hospital for treatment of recurrent, end-stage ovarian cancer. For ten long years she had battled her disease, managing to raise two adopted children, travel extensively through Europe, and supervise the building of her family's home on Cape Cod. "I've lived a full life and tried never to let cancer stop me from fulfilling my dreams," she told me. "In the end, if my illness gets the better of me, I know I've done my best to be happy."

As survivors, we all wish for a long and satisfying future, free of cancer and other disease. But, like anything in life, there are no guarantees. After cancer, many of us come to realize that happiness is not just a state of mind, it's a state of being. It can't be measured by how much money we have or how much power or success we've accrued. Instead it comes from the meaningful activities and enriching relationships we enjoy and how positive we're able to feel about ourselves.

Inevitably there will be days when the stresses and struggles of life leave us frustrated and uncertain. Still, whether you let them get you down is really up to you. Over my fifteen years in practice, I've seen women with the very best of prognoses spend years of their life saddened and depressed, and I've seen others with terminal disease who remain upbeat and hopeful to the end. Overall, however, it's the optimists who seem to stay healthier and get fewer illnesses.

Is there some special secret to their happiness? Perhaps it's their vision to see each day as precious or their ability to find a unique purpose to their life. Sure, they have their low moments. All of us do. Yet in the end they've learned to focus on other people's needs as well as their own and come to see that happiness is not so much getting what they want as it is wanting what they have.

Eleven

FEAR OF RECURRENCE AND SECOND CANCERS

Once a woman has suffered through the rigors of treatment and faced the prospect of her own mortality, the fear of battling cancer again is almost too frightening to consider. Yet in the back of every cancer survivor's mind is the terrifying possibility that one day the disease will return. That's why many survivors tend to panic whenever some new bump or lump surfaces or they experience a small ache or pain.

I know I did. When my own therapy ended, I vowed to take better care of myself, to eat more nutritiously, and to squeeze some form of physical activity into my busy schedule. But if I exercised too vigorously and felt sore the next day, I didn't think muscle strain, I thought the disease had spread to my bones. If I overate at a meal or had that rare piece of chocolate cake, it wasn't indigestion I felt later that evening, it was liver metastasis.

Over time I've learned to turn down the volume on my internal alarm system and balance my fears of recurrence with a healthy dose of self-confidence. But like all survivors, I still feel some degree of anxiety that my cancer might resurface, especially when the time comes each year to visit my own oncologist for follow-up.

None of us likes to have our bodies examined and scrutinized for cancer or to experience those uneasy moments waiting for test results to come back. Each time I hear my doctor's secretary on the other end of the phone, a hole opens up in my stomach as I wait for news that all's well, at least this time around. I see that same fear in my patients' eyes and sense their concern when they come in for annual checkups. Though each of us learns to cope with the fear of recurrence in our own private way, we all know that when it comes to cancer, there are never any guarantees.

Why Cancer Recurs

Why cancer recurs in some women and not others is still somewhat of a mystery, but experts theorize that the process starts when microscopic cells that were not killed off by the original therapy somehow survive by breaking off and drifting to a distant site, lying dormant until just the right combination of risk factors retriggers their growth.

Not every cancer cell that escapes from the original tumor is able to grow elsewhere. Most are stopped by the body's immune system or destroyed by treatment. Yet every cancer differs in its ability to recur and in the places where it may recur. For that reason, recurrent cancers are classified by location: local, regional, or metastatic.

Local recurrence means that the cancer has come back in the same place as the original cancer. It also means there is no sign of cancer in nearby lymph nodes or other tissues. A woman who has had a lumpectomy could later have a local recurrence of breast cancer in or around the area of her surgery.

Regional recurrence means that cancer has begun to grow in the lymph nodes or tissue near the original site but with no evidence of more distant spread. A survivor of cervical cancer, for instance, might have a regional recurrence in the lymph nodes of her pelvis.

Metastasis means that cancer has spread to organs or tissues separate and distant from the original site. For example, an ovarian cancer patient may have metastasis of her disease onto other organs of her abdomen like the liver or diaphragm.

There's no telling if or when cancer will recur. Some survivors never face the return of their disease, while others develop recurrent cancer months, years, or even decades later. I've had patients who were cured of ovarian cancer with six cycles of treatment and others whose tumors withstood the most powerful doses of chemotherapy, resurfacing as full-blown metastases weeks after completion of treatment. The point is, no one knows why some cancers are cured and not others or why some recur within months and others only after years of good health. But no matter what the cause, the key to survival is always early detection, for the sooner cancer is spotted and treated, the greater the chance a woman has to be cured or go back into remission.

By now you are probably asking, "What is my *own* chance for recurrence?" Once again, it's hard to say. Every cancer reacts differently to treatment, and it depends largely on the stage at which your cancer was first diagnosed, its cell type, and your own particular risk factors for disease. Doctors do know that certain types of cancer have a higher rate of recurrence than others and tend to redevelop in specific parts of the body.

Women who have had early (stage one) cervical cancer, for instance, have an 85 percent cure rate five years after treatment with surgery or radiation—in other words, a 15 percent chance of recurrence. Because cervical cancer usually recurs in the pelvis, doctors caution patients to have frequent follow-up pelvic examinations and stay alert for signs of bleeding or pain. But only in rare cases does a cervical cancer spread to more distant regions of the body.

On the other hand, stage one breast cancer (a small tumor with no spread to nearby lymph nodes) carries a 30 percent chance of recurrence after ten years, meaning cancer will be reactivated in three out of ten women within ten years after treatment. That's why many doctors now advocate additional treatment with chemotherapy to decrease the recurrence of breast cancer to 15 percent.

Still, it doesn't mean a woman should ignore her health because she has a low chance of recurrence. Once again, picking up an early recurrence is a woman's best chance for survival. The sooner a cancer is detected, the greater the chances it can be treated before it spreads to other tissues or organs in the body. That's why it is critical that women continue to visit their oncologist and gynecologist for regular cancer screening—to detect not only possible signs of recurrence, but any symptoms of new second cancers as well.

Second Cancers

After you've had cancer once, your risks of developing a second cancer are increased. Studies show that while the majority of cancer survivors remain free of their initial disease, their chances of developing another cancer is about three times higher than the normal population. Sometimes a second cancer occurs because certain individuals carry genes that predispose them to a hereditary cancer syndrome. One syndrome can cause ovarian and breast cancer; another, either ovarian, endometrial, and/or colon cancer. Recently I operated on a fifty-four-year-old accountant named Eleanor for early-stage endometrial cancer. By performing a full hysterectomy, I was able to cure her of uterine cancer. Yet because of her genetic makeup and high-fat diet, she still carried a high risk for colon or breast cancer. To prevent further disease, she would need to be diligent about losing weight and beginning to exercise. Regular screening for early detection of second cancer was also crucial, and I advised she get yearly mammograms, perform monthly self-exams, and follow the American Cancer Society recommendations for sigmoidoscopy.

Ironically, second cancers also may occur because of the type of treatment needed to eradicate the first cancer. Certain alkylating drugs used for chemotherapy can potentially cause a variety of secondary cancers, including leukemia and bone cancer. There is also evidence that the mantle irradiation to the head, neck, and chest area received by Hodgkin's disease survivors may later produce leukemia, bone and soft-tissue sarcomas, non-Hodgkin's lymphoma, skin cancers, and cancers of the thyroid, lung, breast, head, and neck.

In addition, new research shows that breast cancer survivors are at higher risk for Hodgkin's disease. It has been postulated by one well-known investigator that this may occur because as lymph nodes try to protect the body from breast disease, they grow at a faster rate, driving themselves into a mutated and cancerous state that may lead to Hodgkin's lymphoma. Why does this happen in breast cancer and not in other malignancies? We're still not sure. But it may be because some tumors, especially breast cancer, are more prone to lymphatic spread and lymph node involvement than others.

Studies also indicate that women who survive cancer in one of their breasts face two to three times the average chance of developing it in the other breast. In the past it was thought that radiation treatment for the first cancer might be a factor. But new findings from the National Cancer Institute show that radiation treatment for breast cancer contributes very little to the risk of developing a new cancer in the opposite breast. An increased risk in association with radiotherapy is evident only in women who undergo treatment before age forty-five. As a consequence, doctors are now taking special precautions to shield the healthy breast from radiation when younger women are treated for breast cancer.

Still, any survivor who has had radiation for cancer needs to be cautious. Because the risks of later complications persist for more than twenty-five years after treatment, it's critical that every woman perform regular monthly breast exams and be alert for other symptoms of disease. I recently saw a sixty-eight-year-old attorney named Leslie whom I'd treated fifteen years earlier for uterine cancer. Over the years, when she'd come in for checkups, Leslie was careful to point out suspicious moles or lumps that she worried might be cancer. None turned out to be precancerous growths. But at her last checkup I detected a hardening of tissue in her left breast that I suspected might be dangerous.

"When it turned out to be cancer, all I could think about was cutting as much of it out and being rid of the problem," says Leslie, who opted for a mastectomy and immediate reconstruction using tissue from her abdomen. "I could have gone with a less invasive form of treatment, I suppose. But once you've had cancer twice, you become a bit more aggressive about your health."

Most secondary cancers can be treated successfully if detected early. But in order to get thoroughly screened, a cancer survivor needs to know exactly what type of medication or dosage of radiation she received and make certain any potentially endangered organs are checked. For instance, if your chest or neck were irradiated after lumpectomy, be sure your oncologist regularly checks your heart, lungs, and thyroid. If you had a childhood cancer like Wilms' tumor or Hodgkin's lymphoma, make certain your physician thoroughly examines your breasts and prescribes annual mammography screening. It is also important to know what kinds of chemotherapy you were treated with. This information allows your doctor to customize your follow-up exams. Every survivor has the responsibility to be a partner in her own health care, especially when her life and well-being are at stake.

Avoiding Future Cancer

There's no way to completely eliminate your risk for recurrence and second cancer—but taking precautions to avoid certain risk factors makes good sense. Although I've stressed these steps before, it's important to stress them again.

• *Stop smoking*. Tobacco-caused lung cancer will soon become the number one killer of women in this country, accounting for more than three hundred thousand deaths a year. Quitting immediately reduces this risk, with studies showing that women who stop (among those who would have developed cancer because of smoking) increase their life expectancy by as much as *fifteen years*.

• *Stay out of the sun*. Research shows that unprotected sun exposure contributes to a half million cases of nonmelanoma skin cancer each year. Sunburns and tanning are also risk factors for the deadly form of skin cancer called melanoma, the fastest-growing malignancy among women under fifty. The safest way to avoid skin cancer is to avoid sunlight and always to use sunscreen—with a sun protection factor (SPF) of at least fifteen—when you go outside.

• *Eat a low-fat, high-fiber diet*. Diets high in fat, which often include salt-cured, smoked, or pickled foods, may be potentially hazardous.

To minimize your risks, try to eat five to six fruits and vegetables daily, include lots of fiber-rich foods in your diet, and keep your fat allowance below 25 percent of your total calorie intake daily.

• *Limit alcohol.* Heavy drinkers are at increased risk for cancer of the breast and cancers of the larynx, throat, esophagus, and liver. Evidence also shows that alcohol can increase the loss of calcium through your stool and urine and may exacerbate hot flashes during menopause. So drink alcohol in moderation, if at all. Two twelve-ounce bottles of beer, two shots of spirits (eighty proof), and two glasses of wine (eight ounces each) all provide one ounce of alcohol per day. Alcohol consumption averaging more than one to two ounces daily is associated with increased risk to your health.

• *Know the risks of hormone therapy.* The use of estrogen during and after menopause poses an increased risk for endometrial and breast cancer. Before you begin hormone replacement therapy, thoroughly discuss its dangers and benefits with your oncologist and investigate alternative remedies you might try first.

• *Get active.* Studies show that women who consistently exercise three to four times a week appear to be at reduced risk for cancers of the breast, colon, and reproductive system, the three most common types of cancer in women. Exercise also can alleviate hot flashes during menopause.

Screening for Cancer

Eventually the day will come when a universal blood test is available to identify microscopic cancers long before they are visible on X-rays, in sonograms, or by direct endoscopic examination. Already scientists at Johns Hopkins University have begun clinical trials on just such a test to determine whether it actually detects cancer earlier than standard screening methods and, if so, whether earlier diagnosis would improve therapy and survival rates.

There also has been great progress on the genetic level. The gene responsible for a hereditary form of breast cancer that may also put women at an elevated risk for ovarian cancer has been pinpointed, and in time a blood test may be available to screen women at high risk for breast and other types of cancer, allowing them to take preventative measures and potentially avoid the disease altogether. However, it is estimated that this gene is responsible for only about 5 percent of all breast cancers.

So for now, vigilant screening is the best tool survivors have to ensure that a recurrence or second cancer is spotted early enough, when the chance of cure is highest. As you read through the following guidelines, pay careful attention to the warning signs and screening tests for your type of cancer. But also remember that once you've had cancer, you're at higher risk for other forms of the disease as well. A positive result on any of the screening tests does not necessarily mean you have cancer, but it may indicate a need for more testing. The section on pages 197–199 will also give you a clearer idea which tests you'll need on a regular basis to thoroughly monitor your health.

Breast Cancer

Breast cancer is the second leading cause of cancer deaths in American women, but up to 90 percent of women whose breast cancer is found and treated early will survive. Early detection means staying alert for warning signs and following the guidelines for regular screening. If a cancer is caught early, less extensive surgery can be used, often saving the breast itself.

Warning Signs of Recurrence

Any of the following symptoms should be reported to your doctor immediately:

- any lump or thickening in the breast
- swelling, redness, or heat in the breast

- bleeding, discharge, scaling, or retraction of the nipple
- change in breast shape

Signs of advanced disease:

- bone pain
- persistent cough
- weight loss
- mental changes or confusion

Risk Factors

You are at an increased risk of breast cancer if you have a past history of breast cancer; are over the age of fifty; have never had children, had your first child after thirty, or never breast-fed; are more than 40 percent over your ideal weight; or are from a family in which there is a history of premenopausal breast cancer in mothers and sisters.

Additional risk factors include:

- early menarche (before age twelve)
- late menopause (after fifty-five)
- radiation exposure to chest area
- breast biopsy showing atypical hyperplasia
- history of ovary, colon, and/or endometrial cancer
- DES taken during pregnancy
- hormone usage
- high-fat diet
- alcohol use

Screening

Early detection is a critical part to curing and surviving breast cancer. Follow these guidelines to protect your health.

- *Perform monthly breast self-exams (BSE).* Sixty to 70 percent of all breast cancers are found by women themselves. Make it a habit to check your breasts thoroughly at least once a month. BSE should be done the week following your menstrual period or the first day of every month if you are no longer menstruating.

THE MONTHLY BREAST SELF-EXAMINATION

When it comes to breast cancer, early detection can make all the difference. That's why it's essential you examine your breasts every month using these guidelines:

- *In the shower,* with fingers flat, gently slide your hands over every part of both breasts, checking for any lump, hard knot, or thickening.
- *Lying down,* place a pillow under your right shoulder and put your right hand behind your head. Using your left hand, with fingers flat, press gently in a small circular motion, starting at the outermost top edge of your breast and spiraling toward the nipple. Repeat with the left breast. Then check your underarm area—which is also breast tissue—using the same circular motion.
- *Before a mirror,* with arms at your sides, then with arms raised overhead, check for changes in the size, shape, and contour of each breast. Look for swelling, dimpling, or changes in skin texture. Gently squeeze both nipples and look for any discharge.
- *Report any changes* immediately to your doctor. Only about one in ten lumps that premenopausal women report to doctors turns out to be malignant. But your best defense against breast cancer is to know for sure.

- *Have your breasts examined by your oncologist or gynecologist at least once a year.* Usually your doctor will examine your breasts and underarms as part of a routine annual checkup. If you've had breast cancer or a history of suspicious lumps, your physician may recommend more frequent exams.
- *Get a regular mammogram.* Your doctor may advise you to have one every six months if you have had a breast cancer, in order to monitor you more closely the first five years after treatment. A mammogram can detect tumors long before they can be felt. Although there is controversy over when to start being screened for breast cancer, I think it is wise to have a baseline by age forty that will serve as a point of comparison for any later changes in the breast. As an oncologist, I believe that after age forty you should have a mammogram every other year and annually after age fifty unless you have had breast cancer. The frequency of mammograms should be determined by your own cancer history and that of your family, and you should discuss it with your individual physician.

A complete mammogram involves four views, two per breast; the total X-ray dosage ranges from 0.2 to 0.3 rads—only slightly more than that of an average series of dental X-rays. Thanks to advancements in equipment and X-ray film sensitivity, the amount of radiation used in today's mammograms is extremely low and causes no physical harm. Even for younger women, whose denser breasts require a bit more exposure than the fattier breasts of women over fifty, the risk is negligible, if it exists at all.

It must be stressed, though, that mammograms are not a substitute for monthly breast self-exams. No diagnostic test is 100 percent accurate, and cancers are sometimes detected by self-examination that are missed by mammograms. Studies show that 10 percent of breast cancers are not detected, either because the mammogram was not done properly, the equipment (usually the processor that develops the film) was faulty, the lesion itself is of a type that does not show up easily on film, or the radiologist simply missed the signs. Image quality can also depend on the size of the cancer and the type of breast a woman has: a tiny but dense lesion in young, dense tissue may be invisible because of lack of contrast. Also, make certain the center performing your mammography uses machines designed specifically for mammography. Only a registered technologist should take your mammogram, and only a board-certified radiologist should interpret it. The facility should also display an accreditation certificate by the FDA, meaning it goes through yearly inspections and meets strict federal guidelines for quality care.

Prevention

• *Tamoxifen*. The nonsteroidal, antiestrogen drug tamoxifen has long been used to treat postmenopausal women who have had breast cancer and to prevent recurrence and growth of second cancers in the healthy breast. It is important that women taking tamoxifen get regular gynecologic screening, since some research shows an increased incidence of endometrial cancer among patients taking the drug. There is also evidence that tamoxifen may possibly have benefits in preventing osteoporosis and heart disease. More information on its risks and benefits will be forthcoming from a large-scale study of the drug now under way at the National Cancer Institute. Due for completion in the late 1990s, the study will determine tamoxifen's potential role as a preventative drug for healthy women at high risk for breast cancer.

• *Fenretimide (retinoic acid)*. A synthetic, nontoxic derivative of vitamin A, fenretimide is part of a group of compounds called retinoids that are being studied as preventative drugs against breast cancer. Because retinoids naturally regulate the growth of epithelial cells, they may have the potential for controlling abnormal cell growth in other tissues like the breast. Though still unavailable for general use in the United States, a breast cancer survivor may want to investigate becoming part of a clinical study on retinoids through a major medical center. She also should stay current on the medical literature so that when retinoic acid becomes available, she can avail herself of this preventative therapy if it is found to be effective.

• *Prophylactic mastectomy*. To prevent breast cancer, some women from high-risk backgrounds are taking the drastic step of having their healthy breast(s) removed before any cancer is detected. Although such surgery has been performed since the 1970s, it remains highly controversial. In some cases women have had what's known as a subcutaneous mastectomy, where the breast tissue is removed through a small incision, but the nipple and surface skin is left intact; a saline implant or transferred muscle is then inserted to restore the appearance of the breast. But this method still leaves behind enough breast tissue for a cancer to grow. To effectively deter breast cancer, a more extensive and disfiguring operation is needed to fully remove the breast, skin, nipple, and adjacent lymph nodes. This is major surgery for a disease that if caught early, is highly curable. Because of the many risks and costs associated with prophylactic mastectomy, the decision can be made only once a woman has consulted several respected oncologists and fully explored her personal risks for breast cancer as well as other means of prevention like tamoxifen and retinoic aid, when available.

Uterine (Endometrial) Cancer

Cancer of the endometrial lining is the most common reproductive cancer. It most often occurs near menopause and, if caught early, has a 75 percent chance of being cured.

Warning Signs of Recurrence

- vaginal bleeding or discharge
- back pain
- mental changes or confusion
- persistent cough
- weight loss

Risk Factors

Uterine cancer most often occurs in women after age fifty; in women who have never had children or who have had difficulty conceiving; in women who are more than 40 percent over their ideal weight; or in women who went through late menopause. Other risks include:

- use of estrogen replacement therapy
- diabetes, hypertension
- personal history of breast cancer
- family history of colon, breast, endometrial, and/or ovary cancer

Screening

- *Pelvic and rectal exams.* An annual examination by your physician should include a Pap smear and a bimanual exam, in which the doctor feels for abnormalities in the uterus, followed by a rectal exam. Currently no other screening tests are available.

Prevention

- *Oral contraceptives.* In the future, taking oral contraceptives may be a way to prevent uterine cancer. A study by researchers at Boston University and the Harvard School of Public Health indicates that women over fifty who took oral contraceptives for more than a year at any time in the past had 50 percent less risk of developing endometrial cancer than women who never took birth control pills. While research has shown that birth control pills reduce the risk of endometrial cancer, this is the first study to show that their protective effects continue after menopause, when the disease most often occurs.

Ovarian Cancer

Although ovarian cancer ranks second in incidence among gynecologic cancers, it causes more deaths than any other cancer of the female reproductive system. Often the disease is "silent," showing no obvious signs or symptoms until late in its development. Nor are there any truly reliable screening tests for early detection. However, when ovarian cancer is found early, its cure rates are as high as 85 percent. The key to survival is a thorough understanding of your risks, vigilant attention to the warning signs of disease, enrollment in a supervised screening program, and the possible use of preventative therapy.

Warning Signs of Disease or Recurrence

- indigestion
- bloating after meals
- enlarging abdomen (ascites)
- abdominal discomfort or pain
- weight gain/weight loss

Risk Factors

Ovarian cancer most often occurs in women over fifty; in women who have never had children, had their first child after age thirty, who began menstruating early or had late menopause; and in women from families in which there is a history of ovary, breast, colon, endometrial, and/or prostate cancer. Other risks include:

- higher economic status
- fertility drug usage
- high-fat diet

Screening

Because there are still questions about the effectiveness of screening for ovarian cancer, a woman needs to thoroughly discuss with her physician how much risk she carries for the disease (her family's cancer background, her own personal cancer history) before electing to undergo pelvic sonography and tumor marker tests for the disease.

- *Annual pelvic examination.* The pelvic exam is a check of the female organs. The doctor, using a gloved finger and a small instrument called a speculum, checks the vagina, uterus, and ovaries for any sign of a problem. However, the deep-seated position of the ovaries often makes it very difficult for a physician to guarantee that a woman is cancer-free during a regular gynecologic exam.
- *CA-125 blood test.* This tumor marker test looks for certain proteins shed by malignant cells. However, it is not always reliable—in about half of all cases of very early cancer, the CA-125 comes back negative. Some women also have intrinsically high CA-125 results despite having no cancer.
- *Transvaginal color-flow Doppler.* This state-of-the-art sonography is used to spot early ovarian cancers, as well as areas where new blood vessels and changes in blood flow are developing to feed fast-growing cancer cells. However, ultrasound still produces a high rate of false positives, since it can't always distinguish between harmless masses and cancer.

Prevention

- *Oral contraceptives.* Thus far, birth control pills may be one of the only ways of lowering your risk for ovarian cancer. There is evidence that the very act of ovulating—when the surface lining of the ovary breaks open to release an egg—increases the risk for ovarian cancer. In a theory known as incessant ovulation, doctors postulate that the more times a woman ovulates in a lifetime, the more often that break has to heal, and it is in healing, rapidly growing tissue that cancers have their inception. Studies have shown that after five years of continuously taking birth control pills to arrest ovulation, a woman can reduce her ovarian-cancer risk by as much as 60 percent.
- *Tubal ligation.* By their nature, women are constructed so that their insides are connected to the outside world so that sperm can

reach the egg and be fertilized for reproduction. However, other pathogens and carcinogens also have equal access to the womb. If a cancer-causing agent reaches the ovaries, over time it may be able to cause a tumor to grow. In theory, when a woman's fallopian tubes are cut or tied off, this route of transmission is severed. Tubal ligation may also limit blood flow to the ovaries or induce hormonal changes that inhibit development of cancer. Whatever the reason, recent studies show that women with tubal ligation have significantly less (one-third) rates of ovarian cancer than those who don't. For this reason, having your tubes tied after your family is complete may have a preventative effect on ovarian cancer, but we're still not certain to what extent, let alone at what age, the procedure needs to be done to have the greatest benefit.

- *Prophylactic oophorectomy (preventative ovary removal)*. In theory, removal of the ovaries would seem to eliminate the site for ovarian cancer to grow. However, there have been several cases of women whose ovaries were removed and who later developed a type of cancer in their abdomen that was indistinguishable from ovarian cancer. Moreover, if a woman below age forty-five has her ovaries removed prophylactically, she may need to go on estrogen replacement therapy to forestall the effects of osteoporosis and heart disease. Since long-term estrogen has been strongly linked to uterine cancer and also to breast cancer, an oophorectomy in a premenopausal woman may end up substituting one disease for another. However, women from families with hereditary ovarian cancer syndromes may have as high as a 50 percent lifetime risk for ovarian cancer. Before making the difficult decision to have your ovaries removed, you need to thoroughly discuss the procedure's benefits and risks with a gynecologic oncologist.

- *Eliminate use of talc*. Researchers at Harvard Medical School have found that women who use talcum powder on the genital area or sanitary napkins have double the risk of ovarian cancer than those who don't. This finding is controversial, and more research is needed. Particles of talc also have been found in normal ovaries as well as in cancerous ones, suggesting to some investigators that talc may increase a woman's risk. Until more research is done to confirm these findings, the best advice is not to use any form of dusting powder after the bath or on sanitary napkins or diaphragms.

- *Eat a diet low in dairy products.* Yogurt, cottage cheese, and other types of cheese (even the low-fat variety) contain a sugar called galactose, which research suggests may be linked to ovarian cancer in women. The best advice: Drink plenty of skim milk instead to supply the necessary amount of calcium.

Cervical Cancer

Once a disease of older women, preinvasive cervical cancer (also called cervical dysplasia) is now on the rise among women under fifty. If these lesions go undetected and untreated, they can progress to cervical cancer. With early detection, however, most cervical cancer deaths are preventable. Treatment includes surgery and/or radiation therapy.

Warning Signs of Recurrence

- vaginal bleeding or discharge
- back pain
- leg swelling
- weight loss

Risk Factors

Cervical cancer occurs most frequently among women of color; in women who began having sexual intercourse before age eighteen or who have multiple sex partners; in women with less education, regardless of race; and in women past their childbearing years. Other risks include:

- recurrent vaginal warts (human papilloma virus)
- smoking
- failure to have regular gynecologic exams

Screening

- *Pap smear.* Done during a pelvic examination, a Pap test involves the gentle removal of cells from the cervix. These cells are then analyzed under a microscope for abnormalities. The American College of Obstetricians and Gynecologists recommends a yearly Pap screening; if three consecutive tests prove negative, then a woman and her physician can discuss the intervals at which she should be tested.

Prevention

- *Insist on condom use.* Studies show that women with multiple sex partners have less chance of developing cervical cancer when they limit their exposure to sexually transmitted diseases by using condoms.
- *Yearly pelvic exam and Pap smear,* until three negative tests are performed; after that, your interval for examinations will be based on your risk factors.

Colon and Rectal Cancer

Colon cancer is the third most common cancer in women. Early detection is crucial for increasing your chance of survival: if a malignancy is detected in an early, localized stage, the five-year survival rate is about 90 percent. If cancer has spread regionally or invaded adjacent organs or lymph nodes, the survival rate drops below 60 percent. Since three-fourths of colon cancer develops from adenomatous (precancerous) polyps, the goal of screening is not only to detect cancer, but also to monitor for polyps, which can be removed and prevent further disease.

Warning Signs of Recurrence

- gas pains, bloating, cramps, or other abdominal pain
- nausea and vomiting
- blood in stool
- diarrhea or constipation (change in bowel habits)

Risk Factors

Colorectal cancer occurs most commonly in women with a history of colon polyps; in women with a personal or family history of colon cancer or polyps of the colon or rectum; in women who have inflammatory bowel disease or chronic ulcerative colitis.

Other risk factors include:

- high-fat and/or low-fiber diet
- family history of breast, ovarian, uterine, and/or prostate cancer

Screening

- *Stool sample.* Blood in the stool can be a symptom of colon or rectal cancer. There are simple kits available for the collection of stool at home. You'll need to take samples of your stool for three days and avoid certain foods and medicines during that time. Samples can then be mailed or delivered to the doctor's office for examination.
- *Rectal exam.* An examination of the rectum with the doctor's gloved finger can detect rectal tumors.
- *Sigmoidoscopy.* A long, narrow, flexible instrument with a lighted scope on the end is inserted into the rectum to check the rectum and part of the sigmoid colon for traces of colon or rectal cancer. Unlike the stool test, this examination could identify precancerous changes or growths (polyps) that would alert your physician to observe you

more closely. The American Cancer Society recommends a sigmoidoscopy every three years after age fifty. Colon cancer is too prevalent to be ignored, especially if it runs in the family or you've already had a related cancer like breast, uterine, or ovarian cancer.

• *Colonoscopy*. Unlike a sigmoidoscopy, this endoscopic examination examines the full length of the colon on its right and left sides. Since several types of genetic colon cancer seem to strike the upper right portion of the colon, this is the only screening test available that thoroughly checks for polyps in women with a genetic tendency for the disease. Women at higher than average risk should have their entire colon examined annually by colonscopy.

• *Genetic testing*. About one in seven thousand Americans suffer from a genetically inherited form of colon cancer called familial adenomatous polyposis syndrome, and two to three times as many are thought to be at risk of having the disease. Scientists at Johns Hopkins School of Medicine have developed a blood test that detects whether a person has inherited the gene for this disease, in which the lining of the colon sprouts hundred or thousands of tiny, wartlike growths. If left untreated, the condition almost invariably leads to colon cancer, often when patients are in their twenties or thirties and sometimes even younger. Researchers anticipate that a blood test will soon be available at specialized medical centers. But be aware, familial adenomatous polyposis accounts for only about 1 percent of all colon cancers. Researchers have also isolated the gene for a more common form of colon cancer—hereditary nonpolyposis colon cancer—which accounts for about 15 percent of all colon malignancies. A blood test may also soon be available.

Prevention

• *Eat a low-fat diet*. A recent study for colon cancer found that women who get less than one-third of their calories from fat were 50 percent less likely to develop colorectal cancer than those who eat more fat.

- *Increase dietary fiber.* By acting like a scrub brush in the intestines, fiber may help counteract the dangerous effects of fat in the colon, say experts.

Skin Cancer

Close to a million cases of skin cancer are diagnosed each year, primarily in people who have had long-term exposure to sunlight. Most cases are basal cell or squamous cell carcinomas, forms of cancer that need to be removed but are not fatal if treated promptly. However, three-fourths of women who die from skin cancer have malignant melanomas, the fastest-growing form of cancer in young women.

Warning Signs of Recurrence

- mole that bleeds, itches, or hurts; changes in texture; or becomes elevated when before it was flat
- presence of one, or more, large or irregularly pigmented lesions

Risk Factors

Basal and squamous cell skin cancers most often occur in women who are fair skinned, with light hair and blue eyes, and in women who regularly expose themselves to sunlight without skin protection. Melanoma appears to be associated with brief, intense exposures to sunlight and a history of sunburn. Other risk factors for skin cancer include:

- history of previous melanoma
- history of melanoma in a first-degree relative
- three or more blistering sunburns before age twenty
- hormone usage

Screening

- *Examine your skin.* The Skin Cancer Foundation recommends women examine their skin every three months, front and back, with a mirror. Any unusual sore, lump, blemish, or other skin change—especially if it's crusty, scaly, oozing, or bleeding—can be a sign of skin cancer. The "ABCD" rule can help you tell a normal mole from a possible melanoma: A for asymmetry of a mole or growth: melanomas are usually oddly shaped, not round or oval; B for borders that are irregular: the edges of a melanoma are usually ragged, notched, or blurred, not smooth; C for color: skin cancers are often different shades of black, brown, red, tan, white, or blue; D for diameter: malignant lesions are often larger than a quarter inch and continue to grow. If you notice a problem or have a sore that doesn't heal within three weeks, see a dermatologist.

Prevention

- *Stay out of the sun.* Keep time in the sun to a minimum, regardless of the time of year. Wear a long-sleeved blouse and broad-brimmed hat when you're outside; use a beach umbrella when there is no natural shade; don't try to get a tan either by sunbathing or at a tanning salon.
- *Wear sunscreen.* Always use a sunscreen—with a sun protection factor of fifteen or above—when you go outside, even on a cloudy day. Apply to dry skin thirty minutes before going outdoors. Be sure to reapply it every hour, since it can wear off with perspiration or bathing. Don't forget those often missed areas like the lips, behind the knees, and back of hands and ankles, where skin cancers frequently occur.

Regular Checkup Examinations

Even if you do not have symptoms, there are certain tests you should undergo periodically once you reach fifty. Some women ought to get certain tests even earlier. If your doctor does not recommend one of these tests, ask about it. Also, expect your doctor to review test results with you. If you don't hear anything within ten days to two weeks, call.

Pap Test	Every year; after three consecutive normal tests, the Pap test may be performed less often at the physician's and patient's discretion
Mammography	Every one to two years, beginning at age forty; annually after age fifty
Cholesterol	Every two to three years
Fecal Occult Blood Test	Every year
Hemoglobin	Every year
Sigmoidoscopy	Every three to five years after age fifty
Urinalysis	Every year

For the cancer patient, there will also be other blood tests, X-rays, MRIs, and CAT scans that your doctor will specifically order for you based on the kind of cancer you had.

Living with the Threat

One of the frightening things about cancer is its ability to recur months, years, even decades after treatment is complete. That's why cancer survivors tend to live by two key rules: prevention and surveillance. Many of my patients tell me they've become much more aware of their bodies since their cancer and that they've made a conscientious effort to live healthier lives. Rather than wait for cancer to strike again, they've taken action to prevent it: eschewing fatty foods, stopping smoking, building a regular exercise program into their

> **CANCER WARNING SIGNS**
>
> The following are warning signs for the most common cancers in women:
>
> - Lung: a cough that won't go away; coughing up blood; shortness of breath or wheezing
> - Breast: a lump in the breast; a change in breast shape; discharge from the nipple
> - Colon or rectal: changes in bowel habits; bleeding from the rectum; blood in the stool, which appears bright red or black
> - Uterine, ovarian, and cervical: bleeding after menopause; unusual vaginal discharge; enlargement of the abdomen; bleeding or pain during intercourse
> - Skin: a sore that does not heal; a change in the shape, size, or color of a wart or mole; the sudden appearance of a mole
>
> If you have any of these symptoms, contact your doctor immediately. Not every symptom is a sign of recurrence, but when it comes to cancer it's better to be safe than sorry.

lives, and trying hard to get their families to do the same. They make time to get themselves screened regularly for disease, acknowledging that if cancer does strike, they're doing their very best to catch it early.

Of course, there also are women who, once treatment is over, revert to many of the bad habits they engaged in before cancer developed. They give in to the urge to smoke or begin drinking and eating the same unhealthy foods that may have contributed to their cancer in the first place. Perhaps they try an exercise program, but over time they give up on it, finding the effort too draining or cumbersome in their busy lives. There too may be women who find themselves stuck beneath the black cloud of recurrence and who feel so doomed by having had cancer that any effort at prevention or screening seems fruitless.

But ignoring or wallowing in your fears won't make the threat of recurrence go away; denial serves only to mask a problem, not mitigate it. Instead, each of us needs to find some strategy—whether it's through prayer, meditation, visual imagery, professional therapy, or a support group—to gain control of our fears and move on with life. I'm not saying the road back from cancer is an easy one—learning to cope with the unknown never is. But at least, if we make the effort to change our behaviors and minimize our risks, we'll be doing our utmost to stave off disease and perhaps live longer in the bargain. And as survivors of cancer, isn't that what we all truly hope for?

Twelve

JOB AND INSURANCE DISCRIMINATION

*T*he surgery was finished, the scars on her breast were beginning to heal, and though she would still need six to eight weeks of radiation, Lydia's doctor had told her it was safe to return to work and begin getting on with her life. Yet she still felt uneasy.

"I couldn't shake the feeling that everyone would look at me as a victim," says the forty-seven-year-old book editor for a major publishing firm in New York. "I worried that my boss would start limiting my work, or feeding me less prestigious authors to edit. I worried that my insurance benefits would somehow be altered. And I worried that if I wanted to change jobs and advance my career, I wouldn't be able to because I could lose my insurance as a result. Cancer had changed all my options."

Like Lydia, many survivors feel trapped and uncertain about returning to work. There are bills to pay and career goals to consider, yet they wonder if their job choices will still be the same or if they'll have the energy to work as hard as they once did. They also worry about taking off more time for doctors' appointments and further treatment if they need it. And they fear what financial hardship they might face should their disease return in the future.

But going back to work can also have a positive effect. It can bolster our emotional needs as well as our financial well-being, making us feel that we are getting our lives back on track. For many of us, there's a certain need to redirect our focus away from cancer and back to responsibilities and challenges of our careers.

Still, reentry into the workplace is rarely easy. Cancer continues to carry a heavy stigma in our society, and frequently a survivor's return to business may be marred by a spectrum of problems: insensitivity or hostility from co-workers, a demotion in duties or reduction in hours, exclusion from life or disability insurance, and fears of dismissal and loss of benefits.

As a survivor myself, I know firsthand how these pressures can eat away at the carefully rebuilt confidence and inner strength each of us should be permitted to enjoy. Since my own cancer experience, I've been reluctant to consider a job change now that my future is not as secure as it once was. And I kick myself for not signing that life insurance policy I lugged around in my briefcase just weeks before I discovered the cancerous lump in my breast.

But there's no changing the past or the fact that we've had cancer. To our government's credit, the laws are slowly changing to protect cancer survivors against employment and insurance discrimination. Moreover, there has been an increase in the number of financial planners and attorneys available to help women who have had a serious illness like cancer maneuver through the maze of financial obstacles they're likely to face.

Although I can't give you individualized advice or specific strategies to solve your problems, I would like to least offer you a broad overview of your rights and to answer some of the questions you may have about job and insurance issues. That way you can avoid some of the common pitfalls and perhaps find a specialist in your area who can make your return to the well world as smooth and as stress-free as possible.

Facing Your Co-workers

When Rose was diagnosed with breast cancer last year, she kept it a secret from most of her colleagues at work. "I've always been a private person and didn't want a lot of questions about having surgery and chemotherapy, let alone what my chances of survival were," says the forty-six-year-old bookkeeper for a charter bus company. "I suppose I was afraid my boss would see my illness as a form of weakness, so I tried to keep up a good front."

Eventually, however, the treatments took their toll on Rose's health, causing her to lose weight, lose her hair, and suffer from intense fatigue. "One morning, after one of my co-workers found me crying in the bathroom, my supervisor came to talk with me," she says. "When I told him about the cancer, I was terrified I'd lose my job and my health benefits. But the company was wonderful, and helped me take advantage of my short-term disability benefits so I could stay at home and get back my strength."

Often, when a survivor returns to work, one of her predominant concerns is how to face her employer and her co-workers. On the one hand, she may want to share the experiences of her cancer ordeal and find a source of support in the friends she's made at work. On the other, she may want to keep her feelings to herself, fearing her supervisor will treat her differently or think she's incapable of continuing her job responsibilities.

Whether or not you tell colleagues and co-workers about your cancer is a personal decision, and how you deal publicly with your illness is strictly up to you. But there may be practical reasons to discuss your diagnosis, either to get a co-worker to cover for you when you have a doctor's appointment or to ensure you receive appropriate medical benefits. Since you're probably interested in resuming a good working relationship, consider the following suggestions:

- *Plan ahead.* Once your treatments are over, talk to your doctor about returning to work. If she feels you'll need to limit your duties or schedule reduced hours at first, have her outline her recommendations in a note to your employer. Then schedule a frank discussion with your manager or union representative to air your concerns, correct wrong ideas, and decide how best to return to the job.

• *Stay in touch.* Most survivors are surprised by the concern and generosity of their co-workers. When I was home, recovering from treatment, I was flooded with flowers and notes from my staff and colleagues. As my health improved, I made a point to call many of them on the phone, reassuring them of my progress and how I planned to continue my practice. By staying connected, it made my reentry to the job easier and seemed to help my co-workers as well.

• *Share your insights.* Chances are there is someone else in your workplace whose life has been touched by cancer. By sharing your experience and your insights, you can let others like yourself know they are not alone, and it may help lift your own spirits as well.

• *Educate your colleagues.* Many employers have preconceived ideas about a survivor's return to work. They may wonder if the disease will prevent her from being as productive as other workers; whether she can be counted on to stay healthy; what impact her coming back will have on the company's insurance rates; and whether other employees will be fearful or made uncomfortable by her presence.

But when employers learn the facts, they realize many of their beliefs about cancer are unfounded. Numerous studies have found that cancer survivors actually have decreased absentee rates and will usually come to work with minor complaints when other workers would normally stay home. In fact, research shows that most persons who have had cancer work harder, better, and faster than others in order to prove their personal worth on the job.

Also, it's unlikely that one person's illness will affect group insurance costs dramatically, unless the policy covers only a small number of workers. Recently the U.S. Supreme Court ruled that a company, group, or union cannot limit insurance coverage if someone covered by the policy has had cancer or another serious illness.

In order to clarify these issues, you may want to distribute written materials about your type of cancer or invite your doctor or a representative of your local cancer support organization to speak at an informal seminar after work. There they can correct wrong ideas and discuss how newer techniques in screening and treatment have allowed millions of survivors like yourself to live on after the disease.

• *Get help.* If you find that your employer or co-workers' attitudes are getting in the way of your job performance, you should start by talking informally to your supervisor, employee assistance counselor, personnel officer, or union representative. Try to make suggestions for workable solutions: an alteration in your job hours, special equipment in the office, working a day or two from home, or an education seminar with medical professionals. If this fails, you may want to discuss your legal options with an attorney or one of the following agencies in your area:

- The American Cancer Society
- Your state commission on discrimination
- Your state affirmative action office
- U.S. Department of Health and Human Services, Office for Civil Rights
- U.S. Department of Labor, Office of Federal Contract Compliance Programs

Know Your Rights

Though it happens more and more infrequently, some cancer survivors still find themselves discriminated against because of their past medical history. If you feel this is happening to you, be aware of your rights. Under federal and many state laws, an employer cannot treat you differently from other workers because of your cancer background as long as you can do the major duties of your work. If they do, your employer or co-workers may be violating laws that protect you from unfair practices and illegal acts of discrimination.

How Am I Protected?

Under the Americans with Disabilities Act of 1992 (also called the ADA) and the Federal Rehabilitation Act of 1973, a company cannot fire you, demote you or deny you a promotion, or give you an undesirable transfer or alteration of hours if you demonstrate you are capable of doing the job. Nor can an employer require you to take preemployment exams designed to screen for disease or ask you about your health history, unless it affects your current ability to do the job. An employer may ask you detailed questions about your health only *after* you have been offered a job.

Though employers are not required to provide their workers with health insurance, if they do, they must do so fairly. If other coworkers receive insurance benefits, you must, too. Otherwise it could be considered discrimination under federal and state laws. If you have benefits through a group plan at work, a federal law called ERISA prohibits your employer from firing you to prevent you from collecting your insurance.

Are My Family Members Protected, Too?

The ADA also prevents an employer from discriminating against your spouse or another family member because you have had cancer. Several months ago the husband of one of my patients with uterine cancer mentioned he was worried to tell his boss about his circumstances.

"I'm up for a promotion," he told me, "and I probably won't get it if I take time off to care for her after surgery." I agreed to write a note to his employer, outlining the seriousness of his wife's disease and his right by law to fair treatment regardless of her cancer. Two months later he told me his promotion had come through.

Do I Have a Right to Take Medical Leave?

Under a recently enacted federal law called the Family and Medical Leave Act, employers with fifty or more employees are required to provide up to twelve weeks of unpaid, job-protected leave per year for workers who need time off to address their own serious illness or that of a child, parent, or spouse. The law also allows intermittent or reduced work schedule when "medically necessary" (a note from your doctor may be necessary to support this clause). During the leave period, an employer must continue to provide benefits, including health insurance, and restore an employee to the same or equivalent position at the end of the leave. To be eligible, an employee must have worked at least twenty-five hours per week for one year. However, the law does allow companies to exempt their highest-paid workers.

What If I Suffer a Physical Impairment from Cancer?

Federal law and most state laws require an employer to provide cancer survivors with a "reasonable accommodation." An "accommodation" is a change, such as a medical device or altered work hours or duties, that helps you do your job during or after cancer treatment.

After Gloria, a fifty-two-year-old receptionist, underwent chemotherapy for ovarian cancer, she developed partial hearing loss and a severe numbness in both hands. Worried that this would impinge on her ability to answer phones for her company, she went to her supervisor, who agreed to purchase a special phone system. Now she has a headset that raises the volume of incoming calls and an orthotic device that helps her direct calls by hand. In another instance, one of my patients with breast cancer asked her employer to lower the shelving units by her desk and install two-drawer filing units so she wouldn't suffer pain when she raised her arm.

Cancer survivors can also benefit from job accommodations like flexible hours to allow follow-up checkups and subsequent treatment or borrowing sick days from future years. Resources are available to help your employer create the appropriate accommodation for you. Any company, regardless of size, can get free assistance by contacting:

The Job Accommodation Network
President's Committee on Employment of the Handicapped
P.O. Box 468
Morgantown, WV 26505
800-526-7234

Be aware, however, that your employer does not have to make changes that would be an "undue hardship" on the business or on other workers. When Margaret, a sixty-year-old patient with breast cancer, missed a substantial amount of time from her position as a music teacher at a private school, the headmistress was unable to find a temporary replacement for her position and was forced to dismiss her from the job.

"Everyone at the school felt terrible about letting me go, and they've offered to let me come to teach private lessons once my strength begins to return," she says. "But I'd had my job for nearly twenty years, and I'll miss the friends I'd made after all that time."

What Are My Options If Cancer Prevents Me from Doing My Old Job?

While most women are able to return to business as usual after cancer, there may be times when therapy causes a permanent handicap, forcing a survivor to take early retirement or long-term disability leave from work. Readjusting to life with a handicap is never easy, and discovering cancer has cost you your job may further erode your self-esteem and self-image. But though the disease may impair your capability to do one type of work, it can also open up your opportunities to do another. The key is figuring out how best to use your experience and your skills for your future career advantage.

For years Clara had run a cottage industry from her home in Connecticut, selling her hand-knit baby sweaters and accessories to upscale children's stores in New York. But last summer, when she developed breast cancer at the age of forty-nine, a mastectomy caused severe lymphedema in her right arm.

"There was no way I could continue to knit and sustain the business I'd built up, and I felt devastated by my lack of prospects," she recalls. "But I'm not one to give up—the cancer taught me that about myself. So I decided to investigate how I might reconfigure my skills toward a new career."

Clara knew she was good at running a business and had plenty of contacts among wholesalers of wool and knitting goods. She'd also developed unique pattern designs and a score of timesaving knitting techniques. However, it wasn't until she noticed a "For Rent" sign on a storefront near her home that she decided to open a knitting school and woolens shop of her very own.

"I started two months ago, and business has never been better," says Clara. "I've met some wonderful people in my neighborhood, and the work isn't as isolating as it used to be. Frankly, I have to credit the disease for pointing my life in a better direction."

Should cancer alter your own career path, you may find it helpful to discuss your needs with a state vocational/rehabilitation agency. A representative can help you evaluate your rehabilitation potential, give you counseling and guidance on what other types of work you might pursue, and offer placement services. To contact the office nearest you, look in your telephone directory under one of the following state departments: Labor, Human Resources, Public Welfare, Human Services, or Education.

What Can I Do to Avoid Job Discrimination?

If you suspect you're being treated unfairly because of your cancer history, try to work out an informal solution with your supervisor or personnel office before launching into a lawsuit. You want to stand up for your rights, but you don't want to peg yourself as a troublemaker, either. Here are some strategies to consider:

- *Enlist the help of your doctor.* If your employer has doubts about your ability to perform the job, ask your doctor to write a note outlining your continued abilities as well as any restrictions. Often this "expert" advice helps a supervisor better gauge your future productivity and ongoing abilities to do the job. Your doctor may also mention that she's agreed to see you for checkups on, say, late Friday afternoons, so it won't interfere with your work demands.

- *Suggest alternatives.* One of my patients worked out a job-sharing arrangement for several months with a fellow employee on maternity leave. By splitting the hours of the job, each woman was able to take the extra time needed to recover while giving their employer a "full-time" worker in the office.
- *Seek support from your co-workers.* More than eight million Americans are cancer survivors, so it's likely that other workers at your company have had the disease. They too have an interest in protecting themselves from unfair work practices. See if they've had problems in the past and how they rectified the matter. You might be able to pool your ideas for a better working environment.
- *Document the problem.* Make sure you keep a written record of your employment requests and problems. Keep a log of your verbal discussions and the measures you've taken to educate your employer about state and federal antidiscrimination laws. Make complete notes of telephone calls and meetings (including dates, times, and attendees). Also gather together positive examples of your performance at work—written job evaluations, awards, or commendations—that show you are qualified for the job.
- *Talk to a professional.* If you feel you've been treated unfairly because of your cancer history, there are numerous legal remedies you can pursue. However, in most states you must file a complaint within 180 days of the date the discrimination started. If you work for the federal government, you have only 30 days. To save time, you should speak with a lawyer experienced in job discrimination; the National Coalition for Cancer Survivorship (301-650-8868) and some offices of the American Cancer Society (800-ACS-2345) can help you find a lawyer in your area. Alternatively, you can review your case with a representative at your local office of the Equal Employment Opportunities Commission (EEOC); for information, call the EEOC public Information System at 800-669-4000.

What If I Need to Find a New Job?

Looking for a new job can be a nerve-racking experience, especially when you're worried that being a cancer survivor may influence your chances. To present yourself in the best possible way and anticipate any concerns an employer may have, keep in mind these points:

- *Organize your résumé.* An employer is interested in one thing: Are you capable of doing the job? So structure your résumé so it focuses on your skills and experience, not on gaps in your background that may raise questions about your illness and past health problems.
- *Apply for the right jobs.* After cancer, take a hard look at your current skills and capabilities. Then look for jobs you know you can do and at which you'll excel. Employers are perfectly within their rights to reject your application if you show you're not qualified, regardless of your cancer history.
- *Plan for the interview.* Sitting down face-to-face with a prospective employer allows you to impress him with your capabilities and your strengths. You have no legal obligation to discuss your cancer history unless it relates directly to the job you seek. But should the interviewer ask you about your health, don't lie. Instead practice a positive response like "I currently have no medical condition that would prevent me from doing the job well" or "I had surgery for breast cancer three years ago, but I feel fine now and expect to lead a normal and healthy life."

It also may help to bring along a letter from your doctor explaining your current health status. I was happy to do this recently for one of my patients with cervical cancer. In the note I stressed how she was fully recovered from her surgery, was in good health, and had a normal life expectancy.

- *The follow-up.* If you feel you have a good shot at a position, don't hesitate to write or call the employer and reemphasize how much you want the job and will do it well. Should you get an offer, ask to see the benefits package and review it to make sure it meets your needs. In some cases a medical history or physical exam is required before a person can be hired. Check to see if your own physician can perform such an examination to ensure you're not discriminated against because of past health problems.

• *If there are problems.* If you know you're qualified for a job but suspect you weren't hired because of your cancer history, you have a right to take action. First let the employer know that there are antidiscrimination laws to protect cancer survivors. You then may want to contact the local branch of your Equal Employment Opportunities Commission to discuss filing a claim. Remember, however, that legal action can cost you time and money, and it may be more productive to pursue other job opportunities.

Facing Insurance Issues

Once a woman has survived cancer, the need to have adequate health insurance is critical. Not only does the disease make you aware of how costly lifesaving treatment can be, but it also puts you at higher risk for a recurrence or second cancer in the future. As a consequence, a survivor needs to take important steps to maintain "seamless" coverage, to safeguard her assets, and to make certain her medical wishes are adhered to should illness strike again.

Every year the federal and state laws governing insurance coverage continue to change. Increasingly, local governments are taking steps to ensure that *all* individuals have some form of health insurance coverage. Yet thousands of cancer survivors still must contend with the unfair yet legal form of insurance discrimination known as the "preexisting medical condition," which can lock them into jobs they otherwise might leave or threaten their ability to get new or additional coverage in the future.

Until we can get health insurance reform on a federal level, the laws to protect survivors will evolve piecemeal, state by state. As a result, we must be conscientious about keeping up whatever insurance we have, and we must stay informed consumers, learning to advocate on our own behalf.

But figuring out what our own insurance benefits cover and how to take advantage of government-mandated programs can be confusing. And it may be difficult to plan for the possibility of future disease, even death. Still, as survivors of cancer, we must face the catastrophic nature of our illness and take the necessary measures to protect ourselves. In the end, the quality of our lives and the lives of our family could depend on it.

If You Have Medical Insurance, Make Sure You Understand It

One of the harsh realities I faced once treatment had ended was knowing that my options for health insurance had narrowed. So I decided to read up on various state-regulated insurance practices, discovering that my own state of New York has some of the most progressive laws in the nation. By living and working there, I am offered what's known as "portable" insurance. If I hold an individual or group policy covering fifty people or less, I have the right to switch to a comparable policy with another insurance carrier and *not* be denied coverage because of my preexisting illness, providing there is less than a sixty-day lapse between dropping one policy and assuming the next.

This protection is known as "community rating law," and at least twenty states now have similar protective statutes. As of this writing, they include Arkansas, Connecticut, Florida, Hawaii, Kentucky, Louisiana, Maine, Maryland, Minnesota, New Hampshire, New Jersey, New Mexico, New York, North Carolina, Pennsylvania, South Carolina, Vermont, Virginia, Washington, and West Virginia. But before you make any assumptions about your own "insurability," call your state department of insurance and verify how their laws apply to you. Every cancer survivor needs to take a long hard look at the type of insurance she carries and clearly understand its benefits. Otherwise she may not be taking full advantage of what she's paying for—or worse, she may not be as fully covered as she thought. Here are some important points to consider:

- *Understand how your "preexisting illness" affects your coverage.* Altering or switching your health insurance after cancer can be difficult. Many policies carry what's known as a preexisting condition clause—a rule that basically says the company will not cover any costs relating to any condition you had before you became covered by your policy for a certain period of time. Most states have laws governing how long a time that can be. Some say twelve months, some twenty-four months, some as long as five years. And there are even insurance policies that flat-out deny coverage because of preexisting conditions. They specifically say they will not cover cancer-related costs. As horrible as it sounds, many survivors find themselves without adequate health insurance because of this discriminatory exclusion.

Fortunately more and more states are adopting laws that offer some protection against the preexisting illness exclusion through community rating laws and open enrollment periods. To understand where you stand, ask to speak with an examiner at your state insurance department or contact the National Association of Insurance Commissioners about regulations in your area:

National Association of Insurance Commissioners
120 West 12th Street, Suite 1100
Kansas City, MO 64105
816-842-3600
Robert Klein, Director of Research

- *Talk to your benefits manager.* You have a right to know the extent of your job's insurance coverage and that of your spouse. Ask an employee counselor to go over the policy with you, and check to see how long your benefits will last, if they can be limited because of certain medical conditions, if they cover experimental or investigational therapies, and whether they can be taken with you should you terminate your employment. In New York State, for instance, health insurance and disability insurance is portable, and there is usually a thirty-one- to sixty-day window of opportunity during which you can reapply for these benefits.

- *Understand your disability policy.* Some large companies allow you to take your disability policy with you. One of my patients with ovarian cancer worked for a department store with a portable disability policy. When she converted it to an individual policy, she still kept all the benefits of her group insurance. I also treated a woman with breast cancer recently who did not realize her company offered short-term disability benefits. She basically thought that immediately after treatment, despite her pain and fatigue, she would need to jump right back to her job in order to pay her bills. "When I spoke with my supervisor, I found out I was entitled to six weeks of paid disability," says Jane, a fifty-two-year-old bookkeeper. "Now I can let my body heal without worrying that my job's at stake."

- *Has there been a switch in your coverage?* More and more companies are becoming self-insured or switching health care policies, so you need to stay up-to-date on your coverage and make sure the fund's assets are adequate to pay your claims. Chances are you were informed if your firm converted to self-insurance. But state laws vary, and while some require written notification of a switch, others assume you agree to the change unless you object in writing. Make sure you check your bills for changes and read all letters from your insurance carrier carefully.

- *Mistakes happen.* The individuals who process claims at your insurance company are only human, and sometimes they make mistakes. You also may have forgotten to record certain details on your claim, causing it to be rejected. If your insurer denies your claim, first go over the explanation of benefits (EOB) to see what reason they list for not paying. If everything seems in order, make a copy of the EOB and send it back with a request to have your claim reviewed. Fifty percent of the time, claims that are rejected on first submission are paid the second time around. If you need help filing your claims, or cannot figure out a specific problem, try contacting the National Association of Claims Assistance Professionals (708-963-3500).

Your doctor's office staff or the hospital billing department can also help you with the unending piles of paperwork.

• *Learn all you can.* One of the best ways to find out more about coping with insurance problems and how to plan for your finances is to contact your state department of insurance, listed in the Government section of the telephone directory. Local branches of the American Cancer Society may also be able to give you some general but vital details about getting legal advice and coping with insurance obstacles. In addition, the National Coalition for Cancer Survivorship offers a booklet entitled *What Cancer Survivors Need to Know about Health Insurance.* To request a free copy, write the NCCS office at 1010 Wayne Avenue, 5th Floor, Silver Spring, MD 20910; or telephone 301-650-8868.

Getting Insurance If You Lose or Leave Your Job

Thanks to the lobbying efforts of breast cancer survivor Tish Sommers, women who lose their health insurance benefits because of job loss can still preserve their coverage under the federal Consolidated Omnibus Budget Reconciliation Act (COBRA).

A firm of twenty or more employees is required by COBRA to provide you with continuous coverage—regardless of any preexisting conditions—for up to eighteen months if your job was terminated for reasons other than gross misconduct or if your hours were reduced. COBRA also extends to the divorced, separated, or surviving spouse as well as any eligible dependents. If you were eligible to receive Social Security disability at the time your job ended, you can continue COBRA coverage for a total of twenty-nine months. If dependents or a spouse are also on the disability plan, their coverage can go for thirty-six months.

Be aware, however, that COBRA coverage is not free or automatic. If you wish to continue your health insurance under COBRA, you must pay the full premium rate for this coverage, plus 2 percent for administration costs, *and* you must notify your employer *in writing* within sixty days of your desire to use these benefits.

Still, for Lila, one of my patients with ovarian cancer, the choice of paying for COBRA and collecting long-term disability payments from her manufacturing firm was better than leaving her job and trying to find an individual policy while she collected unemployment insurance. "Getting unemployment would have meant I was still willing and able to go back to work, and quite frankly, I simply didn't have the stamina," says the fifty-four-year-old operations manager. "This way, if I need more chemotherapy or radiation, I'm still insured and I continue to collect sixty percent of my salary for the next twenty-nine months."

You may also be able to get additional life insurance from your employer. This may be basic coverage or supplemental coverage. You or your spouse may also be able to get spousal life insurance from each other's employer. Most states allow you to convert the life insurance (without medical proof of insurability) to an individual policy when you leave the employer.

Disability insurance is also another benefit which may be offered from your employer. If you work for a large company, there may be no medical questions to be answered. If you pay the premium, the benefits received under the plan will be tax-free. If the employer pays the premium, the benefits will be taxable. If you're collecting disability for a period of a year, you can take advantage of vocational training programs that allow you to work and collect a paycheck for as long as nine months while you continue to receive your Social Security benefits. This way you can find out if you are strong enough to continue working or should stop altogether and receive Medicare.

As a cancer survivor, you should also know that in certain states like New York, an insurer is required to pay medical costs for up to a year on a disabled person—*even if the policy has been canceled.* I had one patient with recurrent ovarian cancer who was going to be eligible for Medicare as of November 1. However, her Blue Cross/Blue Shield premium was due a month before, on October 1. Her husband did not want to pay the one-month premium while they waited for Medicare, so they canceled the policy. However, in the middle of October my patient's condition worsened, requiring her to be hospitalized and given many costly treatments. Because she developed the "disability" of ovarian cancer prior to losing her insurance coverage, Blue Cross was forced to cover the insurance needs of her cancer treatment. But had she broken her hip, or developed some new disability after the policy ended, Blue Cross would not have covered its treatment.

Another option for getting insurance is to join a health maintenance organization (HMO). Many states offer open enrollment periods when you can be accepted regardless of your health history. Although you will be restricted to using only the HMO's doctors and their hospitals, one recent study showed that women enrolled in HMOs were diagnosed significantly earlier for cancers of the breast, cervix, colon, and skin than fee-for-service patients.

As of this writing, states with open enrollment periods include the District of Columbia, Maryland, Massachusetts, Michigan, New Hampshire, New Jersey, New York, North Carolina, Pennsylvania, Rhode Island, Vermont, and Virginia. To stay up-to-date, check with your state department of insurance to see whether your state has begun offering open enrollment periods.

You also may have an opportunity to obtain group health insurance with a limited waiting period for preexisting conditions through a professional, alumni, membership, or political organization to which you belong. It might also be cost-effective to join such a group in order to get their comprehensive health coverage. Visit your local library and check the *Encyclopedia of Associations* for your areas of interest. Then contact the organizations and ask what types of health, disability, and life insurance they offer to members.

Protecting Your Assets

After cancer, getting back to work and securing your insurance benefits may be your chief concerns. But you also must recognize that you've faced a deadly illness and need to take some necessary steps to reduce your financial burden *and* ensure that certain "crisis" plans are in place should the disease return.

"As a cancer survivor, there are some risks you can buy protection for and others you must plan for," says Patricia Drivanos, a highly respected financial planner who specializes in serious illness. "The bottom line is you have to plan for the worst and hope for the best."

With her help, I've drawn up the following list of protective strategies:

- *Maintain a healthy emergency fund.* These days most people are keeping very small amounts of money in low-interest CDs and money markets, searching instead for higher rates from longer-term investments like Treasury bonds and annuities. But it's smarter to keep at least one year's living expenses in a liquid, low-risk account in case you need it. For instance, rather than a stock market investment, you're safer putting your assets into a bank account or government savings bonds, which can be easily liquidated in an emergency. If you become disabled before age fifty-nine-and-a-half, you also can draw down on your IRAs and 401(k) money without any preterm penalties. Granted, the money is still taxable, but it's available funds you didn't have access to before your illness.
- *Control your cash flow.* Cut out unnecessary expenses, determine the amount needed each month, and know where it is coming from. When you come through a serious illness like cancer, it jolts you into a state of alertness, and you need to plan for the worst-case scenario.
- *Keep up your life insurance coverage.* Many survivors consider eliminating their life insurance premiums as a means to reduce their expenses. However, if the insurance is meant to protect the needs

of your spouse and children, it's more important than ever to keep payments up-to-date. By obtaining what's known as an "in-force ledger" from your insurance company, you can determine if premiums may be stopped or reduced temporarily while keeping the death benefit intact. Even reducing the death benefit and making no payments for a while is a better bet than eliminating life insurance coverage altogether. Also review your beneficiary designations to make sure your life insurance goes to the right people.

Life insurance is not only for beneficiaries, but is an asset that may be accessed if there is a reoccurrence of a serious illness. Funds may be raised from life insurance policy loans, accelerated benefits, and viatical settlements.

If you have permanent insurance, such as whole life, variable life, or universal life, you may have built up a cash value in the policy, and you can request a loan of these funds from the life insurance company. The rate of interest charged is usually lower than other sources of credit, and the loan does not have to be paid back. The loan is deducted from the death benefit when the insured dies.

Accelerated benefits are a pre-death settlement made by the insurance company to the seriously ill and insured. Typically, the life expectancy for such a settlement is one year or less; the requirements and benefits vary by insurance company.

Viatical settlements are the sale of a seriously ill insured's life insurance policy to a third party. For viatical settlements, the life expectancy of the insured should be two years or less. However, some companies will make offers on policies of people with longer life expectancies. The sale price is generally between 60 and 80 percent of the face value of the policy.

- *Look into creditor insurance.* Healthy people would never get insurance on their credit cards—it's an expense they simply don't need. But once you've survived cancer, it may be worth paying $3.40 a month if there's an average outstanding balance of $1,000 on your credit card. Credit card insurance requires no proof of insurability, and if you die or become disabled, it will pay off your balance. This coverage, available through the lender, can also be put on mortgages (usually under $50,000), home equity loans, and car loans. Call the toll-free customer service number on your credit cards, or ask your banker to find out if it is available from your lender. In one instance a patient with breast cancer planned to go out on disability leave. First she bought insurance on her MasterCard, made numerous purchases on credit, and began making minimum payments. When she went on long-term disability, her credit card payments were paid for two years. There's no scam involved with this, just advanced planning. However, if you decide to try this yourself, make sure the credit card is in your own name, not that of your spouse.

- *Establish a trust.* Numerous types of trusts can be set up to avoid the depletion of your assets. Some allow you to manage your own funds until you become disabled; others transfer decision-making powers to a "trustee," who holds title to your property and makes decisions about your assets. Because of the myriad of complicated tax laws, you should consult an attorney who specializes in trusts or estate planning to find out the best way to set aside funds and ensure their proper management should you become ill.
- *Choose a guardian.* Recently one of my patients called me, upset and perplexed. Though her ovarian cancer was in remission, she'd begun to worry about the care of her son should she fall ill in the future. The boy, fifteen, has severe cerebral palsy and requires constant supervision and specialized care. Her husband left her several years ago, and she is the sole breadwinner at home. If her disease comes back, her life—as well as her son's—might be in jeopardy. On my recommendation she met with an attorney, who helped her update her will and designate a family friend as her son's guardian should she die or become too ill to care for him. It wasn't the perfect solution—nothing is when you're faced with choosing someone to care for your children or dependent spouse. But in a small way it put her mind at ease to know he'd be watched over by someone close to the family and not a stranger appointed by the state.
- *Consult a professional.* Understandably, many survivors have a

hard time confronting the eventuality of their death. There's a lot of emotionalism involved, and often it's best to rely on a specialist who can handle these matters in a detached and professional fashion.

Frequently large hospitals and organizations like Cancer Care and the American Cancer Society offer financial-planning seminars for cancer patients and their families. You can also contact the not-for-profit organization Affording Care, the only national group helping the sick manage their personal finance and insurance problems. They provide free seminars for individuals and a list of specially trained financial planners around the country; their address is 429 East 52nd Street, 4G, New York, NY 10022 (phone 212-371-4741).

It also helps to contact an attorney who specializes in estate planning. This way you can set up certain legal documents—a will, irrevocable trust, health care proxy, living will, and/or durable power of attorney—that will allow others to take responsibility for your care and finances should cancer or another medical problem arise. If your own regular attorney does not specialize in estate planning or trusts, you can contact the National Academy of Elder Law Attorneys to help you find a skilled lawyer near your home.

You can also enlist the help of your oncologist. Although your treatments are finished, your physician is still concerned for your health and may be able to ease the financial burden you face. Tell your doctor up front about the extent and type of insurance coverage you have, what the lifetime maximum of the policy is, and which tests require advanced approval. Often, physicians can word a diagnosis in such a way so that necessary screenings tests and procedures are covered under most policies. If you need to go on long-term disability or sell your life insurance to a third party to cover health costs, your doctor can correctly fill out the appropriate forms and give the necessary estimate of life expectancy.

- *Reconsider a divorce.* This sounds like a drastic measure, but if the ordeal of cancer and other problems are leading you toward divorce, you should clearly understand the economic ramifications of your decision. Many women are unaware that if a marriage lasts less than ten years, the retirement benefits of Social Security are based *not* on their husband's earnings, but on their own. Obviously, if your salary is comparable to your husband's or if you've been married only a short time, it may not be worth the emotional stress to stick it out for ten years. But if you've been married eight or nine years, you might find it more financially worthwhile to postpone signing divorce papers until the marriage hits the ten-year mark.

Preserving Our Dignity

We all hope to live a long and happy life after cancer, filled with the joy of watching our children grow and their families prosper and thrive. We want to make plans for the future and work toward our goals, travel to far-off places, or see the world from a cozy seat in our backyard. We'd like to carry on with our days in good health and good spirit. But we also realize how quickly things can change and how one day we may be well and the next day deathly ill.

By this time we're familiar with the rigors of medical treatment and how helpless and bereft of dignity one can feel. And should we face any further battles with cancer or another catastrophic disease, we want it done with as much caring and concern as possible.

That's why it's important now—while we're healthy and able—to take the right steps to protect and preserve our rights. To this end, I counsel all my patients to set up a health care proxy and living will. In certain states like New York, you can appoint a person known as a health care proxy to make medical decisions on your behalf should you become incapable of communicating such decisions to your physician. A living will is slightly different in that it tells what sorts of lifesaving procedures you want or don't want should you become seriously ill.

For help in setting up a health care proxy and living will, contact Choice in Dying, 200 Varick Street, New York, NY 10014 (phone 212-366-5540). They can provide you with proper documents to sign and instruct you on how to keep them on file with your doctor and/or attorney.

Finally, make sure your will is up-to-date and that you have a durable power of attorney in place. Should you need further cancer treatment, you may be too ill to pay your bills on time. And the last thing you need is to find out your health insurance has been canceled because you didn't pay the premiums while you were sick.

Do's and Don'ts of Insurance

To avoid problems with your health insurance, here are some further tips:

- *Don't cancel your current health insurance policy until you have a new one.* In many cases there will be a waiting period for preexisting conditions. Make sure you hold on to your old policy until this waiting period has expired and your new coverage is in effect.
- *Don't lie on your insurance application.* When you apply for a health, disability, or life insurance policy, it's customary for the insurance company to verify the medical details of your application with the Medical Information Bureau (MIB) in Boston, Massachusetts. With its vast stores of computerized data, the MIB can compare your information against other insurance claims that you or a hospital may have filed in the past seven years. If they uncover omissions, misrepresentations, or false health conditions on your application, then may deny your benefits or cancel your policy.
- *Don't buy "cancer insurance."* Some insurance companies have begun offering "cancer policies" that pay benefits *only* on cancer treatment. But most insurance experts recommend against them, and some states have even banned their sale. The premiums are high, the policies often exclude complications from cancer treatment, and if you have a solid basic and major-medical plan, you'll be duplicating your coverage and wasting your money.
- *Do deduct your medical costs.* To supplement your insurance, take all the federal income tax deductions for health care costs you're allowed. Keep a log of your gas mileage for trips to and from doctor

appointments, out-of-pocket expenses for prescription drugs and equipment, and any hotel or meal expenses during lengthy medical visits.

- *Do buy life insurance on other family members.* If the incidence of cancer is high within your family, it may be a good idea for your children to purchase life insurance while they are healthy. One of my patients with breast cancer took out a policy on her daughter when she learned more about the genetic links of the disease: "I wanted to be sure my grandchildren would be taken care of should anything happen to me or their mother."
- *Do get help.* Unraveling the complexities of your insurance options can be a nerve-racking experience. Fortunately there are specialists who can help. Consult your local cancer organization, your social worker, or the resource guide in the back of this book to find professionals who can counsel you about insurance problems and best protect your assets for the future.

· AFTERWORD ·

Where Do We Go from Here?

This morning, as I walked outside and felt the wind blow through my scalp, I rejoiced at having hair. It is such a simple pleasure, feeling it tangle across my forehead and pull against my skin. Everyone wants to know why I'm letting it grow past my ears and toward my shoulders, why I don't seem to care that it looks wild and disheveled at times. For me, there's a need to have it long and styled the way it was before I got sick. My hair has become a symbol of my disease—and once I have it back to the way it was, I will have closed my own personal chapter on cancer—hopefully for good.

As survivors, each of our lives will be different. Yet what we all will share in common is cancer and our victory over a dreaded disease. Together we have overcome a major trauma, and it will take time to rebuild our strength. Sometimes our confidence will falter and we'll wonder how to get through to the next day. But always there will be the joy of seeing a new sunrise and of knowing we are alive to enjoy another day.

· SUPPORT GROUPS AND RESOURCES ·

Support Groups

National Coalition for Cancer Survivorship
1010 Wayne Avenue, 5th Floor
Silver Spring, MD 20910
301-650-8868

   A national support network with a focus on advocacy; also a clearinghouse for survivorship-related information.

American Cancer Society
1599 Clifton Road NE
Atlanta, GA 30329
800-ACS-2345

   Sponsors patient, survivor, and family support and education groups.

Cancer Care
1180 Sixth Avenue
New York, NY 10036
212-302-2400
Long Island office 516-364-8130
New Jersey office 201-379-7500
Connecticut office 203-854-9911

   Free professional counseling and other assistance for survivors and their families; computerized cancer-resource directory.

Cancervive
6500 Wilshire Boulevard, Suite 500
Los Angeles, CA 90048
213-203-9232

Assists cancer survivors to face and overcome challenges of "life after cancer."

Cancer Information Service
National Cancer Institute
800-4-CANCER

Information available in both English and Spanish.

Cancer Guidance Hotline
1323 Forbes Avenue
Pittsburgh, PA 15219
412-261-2211

Links callers with trained volunteers who have experienced cancer.

Cancer Support Network
Essex House, Suite L10
Baum Boulevard at South Negley Avenue
Pittsburgh, PA 15206
412-361-8600

Professional and peer-support network for cancer survivors, families, and friends.

CAN ACT (Cancer Patients Action Alliance)
26 College Place
Brooklyn, NY 11201
718-522-4607

Addresses problems of access to advanced cancer treatments, barriers created by FDA drug approval process, and restrictive insurance reimbursement policies.

National Alliance of Breast Cancer Organizations (NABCO)
9 East 37th Street, 10th Floor
New York, NY 10016
212-719-0154

Provides breast cancer patients and survivors with information on treatment and local support groups; complete breast cancer resource list.

Society of Gynecologic Oncologists
401 North Michigan Avenue
Chicago, IL 60611
312-644-6610/800-444-4441

Resource information on cancers of the female reproductive tract and referral services for oncologists in your area.

Candlelighters Childhood Cancer Foundation
7910 Woodmont Avenue, Suite 460
Bethesda, MD 20814
800-366-2223/301-657-8401

Provides information, support, and advocacy to survivors of childhood cancer and families of children with cancer.

Coping Magazine
2019 North Carothers
Franklin, TN 37064
615-790-2400

The only nationally distributed consumer magazine for people whose lives have been touched by cancer.

National Cancer Survivors Day Foundation
2019 North Carothers, Suite 100
Franklin, TN 37064
615-794-3006

Information on America's nationwide annual celebration for cancer survivors, celebrated the first Sunday in June each year in communities throughout the United States.

Two: *Putting Treatment Behind You*

The Wellness Community
2200 Colorado Avenue
Santa Monica, CA 90404
310-453-2300

Provides free psychosocial support to people fighting to recover from cancer; has fourteen facilities located throughout the nation.

Four: Taking Care of Your Health: Diet, Nutrition, and Lifestyle

American Institute for Cancer Research
1759 R Street NW
Washington, D.C. 20009
800-843-8114

Information on cancer and nutrition, cookbooks and brochures.

National Women's Health Network
1325 G Street NW
Washington, D.C. 20005
202-347-1140

Provides preventative diet information focused specifically on breast cancer.

Five: Coping with Physical Scars

The National Lymphedema Network
2215 Post Street
San Francisco, CA 94115
800-541-3259

United Ostomy Association
36 Executive Park, #120
Irvine, CA 92714
714-660-8624

American Hair Loss Council
800-274-8717

Information and resources on hair loss.

American Society of Plastic and Reconstructive Surgeons
444 East Algonquin Road
Arlington Heights, IL 60005
708-228-9900; 800-635-0635

Information and referrals for reconstructive surgery after cancer.

The Breast Implant Information Network
800-887-6828

Medical and legal information for women with or considering breast implants.

My Image After Breast Cancer
6000 Stevenson Avenue, Suite 203
Alexandria, VA 22304
703-461-9616

Twenty-four hour "HOPEline" staffed by breast cancer survivors to give information and counseling.

Lady Grace Stores
800-922-0504

Chain of post–breast surgery stores; mail order available. Medicare accepted.

SHARE (self-help for women with breast or ovarian cancer)
19 West 44th Street
New York, NY 10036
212-719-0364

Y-ME
National Organization for Breast Cancer Information and Support
18220 Harwood Avenue
Homewood, IL 60430
800-221-2141

Prosthesis and wig bank for women with financial need; will ship anywhere in the United States.

ENCORE
YWCA of the USA
726 Broadway
New York, NY 10003
212-614-2700

Post-treatment program for women who have had breast cancer, consisting of peer support and exercise.

American Brain Tumor Association
2720 River Road, Suite 146
Des Plaines, IL 60018
800-886-2282

Offers free services, publications, support groups, referral services, and a pen-pal program for patients and survivors of brain tumors.

International Association of Laryngectomees
1599 Clifton Road NE
Atlanta, GA 30329
404-320-3333

Let's Face It
Box 711
Concord, MA 01742
508-371-3186

Mutual-help network for the facially disfigured.

Leukemia Society of America
733 Third Avenue
New York, NY 10017
212-573-8484

Services for patients and survivors of leukemia and other hematic cancers.

Six: Sex After Cancer

American Association of Sex Educators, Counselors, and Therapists
435 North Michigan Avenue, Suite 1717
Chicago, IL 60611
312-644-0828

Provides names of registered sex therapists in your area.

The Mautner Project
P.O. Box 90437
Washington, D.C. 20090
202-332-5536

Information, support, and advocacy to lesbians with cancer and their families.

Support Groups and Resources · 235

Xandria Collection
Lawrence Research Group
P.O. Box 31039, Department DP
San Francisco, CA 94131

Good Vibrations
3492 22nd Street
San Francisco, CA 94110

Discreetly packaged catalogs for sexual aids and products.

F. E. Young & Co.
1350 Old Skokie Road
Highland Park, IL 60035

Milex Products, Inc.
Milex-Vaginal-Hymenal Dilators
Chicago, IL 60631

Mail-order vaginal dilators by prescription.

Seven: The Road to Motherhood

Society for Assisted Reproductive Technology
c/o American Fertility Society
1209 Montgomery Highway
Birmingham, AL 35216
205-978-5000

Member society for institutions conducting assisted reproductive procedures.

National Infertility Network Exchange
P.O. Box 204
East Meadow, NY 11554
516-794-5772

Peer support groups for infertile couples, education programs, and referral service.

Gilda Radner Ovarian Cancer Registry
Roswell Park Cancer Institute
Elm and Carlton Streets
Buffalo, NY 14263
716-845-3110

National registry providing information on screening and detection for ovarian cancer.

Hereditary Cancer Institute
Creighton University
P.O. Box 3266
Omaha, NE 68103
800-648-8133; 402-280-2942

Evaluates families for evidence of hereditary cancer, identifies high-risk relatives in cancer-prone families, provides recommendations for early screening and detection.

Eight: Cancer's Effect on the Family

Well Spouse Foundation
17456 Drayton Hall Way
San Diego, CA 92128

Network of support and advocacy groups for families of the chronically ill.

American Association for Marriage and Family Therapy
1100 17th Street NW
Washington, D.C. 20036
202-452-0109

Referrals for family therapists nationwide.

Nine: Facing Menopause

DES Action
1615 Broadway, Suite 510
Oakland, CA 94612
516-775-3450 (East Coast office)
415-826-5060 (West Coast office)

Offers counseling, educational materials, and newsletter about exposure to DES.

Ten: Stress, Loneliness, and Depression

The Humor Project
110 Spring Street
Saratoga Springs, NY 12866
518-587-8770

Free catalog and resources on humorous material; conferences held on use of humor in coping with illness.

Eleven: Fear of Recurrence and Second Cancers

Susan G. Komen Breast Cancer Foundation
5005 LBJ Freeway, Suite 370
Dallas, TX 75244
800-IM-AWARE

Information on screening and treatment for breast cancer.

The Skin Cancer Foundation
Box 561
New York, NY 10156
212-725-5176

Medical education on reducing incidence and mortality of skin cancer.

Strang Cancer Prevention Center
428 East 72nd Street
New York, NY 10021
800-521-9356; 212-794-4900

Provides free national resources for women at high risk for cancer.

Twelve: Job and Insurance Discrimination

U.S. Equal Employment Opportunity Commission
1801 L Street NW
Washington, D.C. 20507
800-872-3362

American Civil Liberties Union (ACLU)
132 West 43rd Street
New York, NY 10036
212-944-9800 (or call local listings)

Provides legal assistance for victims of discrimination.

National Rehabilitation Information Center (NARIC)
U.S. Department of Education
National Institute on Disability Rehabilitation Research
8455 Colesville Road, Suite 935
Silver Spring, MD 20910
800-34-NARIC (voice/TDD)

Information center providing resources and services for the disabled.

President's Committee on the Employment of People with Disabilities
1111 20th Street NW
Washington, D.C. 20036
202-653-5044

Rehabilitation Services Administration
Department of Human Services
605 G Street NW
Washington, D.C. 20001
202-727-3227

Provides general information on vocational rehabilitation programs in your area.

National Insurance Consumer Organization
121 North Payne Street
Alexandria, VA 22314
703-549-8050/help line 800-942-4242

Nonprofit public interest group providing information on health and life insurance.

National Self-Help Clearinghouse
25 West 43rd Street, Room 620
New York, NY 10036
212-642-2944

Information and regional self-help services, particularly on insurance concerns and protection of employment rights.

National Consumer Helpline
800-942-4242

National Hospice Organization
1901 N. Moore Street, Suite 901
Arlington, VA 22209
800-658-8898

Resource information for terminally ill patients and their families.

· INDEX ·

ABCD rule, 197
Abdominal cramps, 78
Acetaminophen, 35, 81
Adenocarcinoma, 119
Adrenal gland, 39
Adriamycin, 78, 79
Aerobic exercise, 52, 53, 54
Affording Care, 222
Alcohol, 183
  abuse, 21, 29
  and calcium, 51–52, 160
  and depression, 173
  and hot flashes, 159
  reducing intake, 37, 47–48
  and second cancer, 181, 194
  and stress, 168
Alkeran, 118
Alkylating drugs, 178
Alpha-methyldopa (Aldomet), 158–59
Alternative treatments
  for cancer, 64
  to hormone replacement therapy, 157–62
Amenorrhea, 118
American Association for Marriage and Family Therapy, 236
American Association of Sex Educators, Counselors, and Therapists, 234
American Brain Tumor Association, 234

American Cancer Society, xiii, 60, 114, 178, 195, 205, 210, 216, 222, 229
American Civil Liberties Union, 237
American College of Obstetricians and Gynecologists, 193
American Hair Loss Council, 232
American Institute for Cancer Research, 232
American Medical Association, 48
American Society of Plastic and Reconstructive Surgeons, 232
Americans with Disabilities Act (ADA, 1992), 206
Androstenedione, 39
Anemia, 32, 86
"Aneuploid" tumor, 126
Anticancer regimens
  alternative, 64–65
  future, 87–88
Antidepressants, 16, 23, 78
Antioxidants, 49–51
Appearance, 8
Appendicitis, 78
Appetite, 31, 173
Arthritis, 31, 54, 74
Artificial sweeteners, 62
Astroglide, 99, 100, 104
Attitudes
  coping tips, 25–26
  and immune system, 19–20

Babysitting, 171
Backache, 31
Basal cell carcinoma, 62, 196
Beans, 43, 46, 64
Behavioral modification, 23, 61
Benjamin, Harold, 20
Beta-carotene, 49, 50
Bile acids, 45–46, 153–54
Biopsy, 2–3
Biphosphanates, 160
Bladder
   and menopause, 144, 147
   reconstruction, 69, 99
Bladder cancer, 48, 49, 50, 60
Bleomycin, 78, 79
Bloating, 31
Blood clots, 153, 158, 161
Blood sugar, 60, 168
Blood tests, 32, 181, 190, 195, 199
Blue Cross/Blue Shield, 217
Body image, 67
   and sex, 89–90, 93–95
   and singles, 109
Body/mind connection, 164–65
Bone
   density, increasing, 159
   loss, monitoring, 152, 156, 160
   pain, 31
   scan, 5, 32
Bone cancer, 178
Bone marrow suppression, 85–86
Bowel regularity, 46
Brain, and radiation, 80
BRCA1 gene, 127
Breast
   and caffeine, 48
   exam by doctor, 185
   reconstruction, 73–76, 95, 110
   removal, 67–68, 73–74, 90
   self-exams (BSE), 184
   stimulation, 107
   See also Mastectomy
Breast cancer, 35
   and alcohol, 47, 48, 181
   and attitude, 164–65
   and diet, 56–57, 64, 65, 155

   discovery and treatment, 1–8
   and exercise, 52, 53
   and fat intake, 38, 39, 40–41
   and fiber, 45
   follow-up care, 28, 32
   and genetics, 127, 128, 181–82
   and hormone replacement therapy, 145, 148–53, 155
   and lymphedema, 84
   and Megace, 158
   physical therapy after, 35
   and pregnancy, 124–26
   and premature menopause, 146–47
   prevention and screening for, 177, 182–87
   and second cancer, 178–79, 188, 194
   and sex, 89, 91–94, 107, 110
   signs of recurrence, 30–31
   and smoking, 60
   tamoxifen therapy for, 161–62
   vitamins, 50
   warning signs, 198
Breast Implant Information Network, 233
Broccoli, 46, 50, 51, 160
Brooks, Mel, 168
Buffered aspirin, 35
Bush, Barbara, 147
Butter substitutes, 43
B vitamins, 48

CA-125 blood test, 190
Cabbage, 46, 50
Caffeine
   and calcium, 51–52, 160
   and cancer, 48–49
   and hot flashes, 159
Calcitonin, 160
Calcium
   in bones, 146, 181
   -rich foods, 51, 192
   supplements, 29, 51–52, 159–60
Calories, 59
   from fat, 42
CAN ACT, 230

Cancer
  beneficial side of, 14–15
  future prevention, 64–65
  future treatments, 87–88
  and heredity, 126–30
  myths about, and sex, 91–93
  pregnancy after, 113–31
  prevention, and lifestyle, 37–64
  prevention and screening for, 180–99
  reason for recurrence, 176–78
  and stress, 164–65
  understanding, 33–34
  warning signs, 198
Cancer antigens, 32
Cancer cachexia, 20
Cancer Care, 222, 229
Cancer Guidance Hotline, 230
Cancer Information Service, 230
"Cancer insurance," 224
Cancer Support Network, 230
Cancer Survivors Day, 130
Cancer survivors
  and coping with scars and side effects, 66–88
  and depression, 172–74
  dignity of, 223–24
  and emotions at end of treatment, 10–15
  and family, 132–43
  and fatigue, 16–17
  and first anniversary, 8–9, 12–13
  genetic legacy of, 126–29
  and hormone replacement therapy, 151–57
  and insurance, 212–18
  and job discrimination, 201–12
  and living with compromise, 86–88
  and loneliness, 169–72
  low-fat diet for, 39
  and menopause, 144–62
  number of, xiii
  and pregnancy, 113–31
  and prevention of recurrence, 175–200
  protecting assets, 218–23
  relationship with children, 138–40
  and role changes, 141–43
  and sex, 89–112
  single, 109–10
  and stress, 165–69
  support groups and therapy for, 23–25
  and uncharted territory, xiii–xiv
Cancervive, 230
Candlelighters Childhood Cancer Foundation, 231
Carcinomatosis, 129
Cardiotoxic medications, 78
Cash flow, 219
CAT scan, 32, 34, 199
Cervical cancer, 60
  and diet, 50
  follow-up care, 32
  and hormone replacement therapy, 154–55
  and pregnancy, 117, 119
  prevention and screening for, 192–93
  and recurrence, 177
  sex after, 90, 98–100
  warning signs, 198
Cervical dysplasia, 64
Checkup exams, 197–99
Cheese, 43, 63
Chemotherapy, 15
  and attitude, 20
  coping with side effects, 76–79, 87–88
  and diet, 46, 57–58
  emotions at end of, 10–13
  and exercise, 53
  and job rights, 207–8
  and mastectomy, 74
  pregnancy after, 116, 118, 127
  and premature menopause, 146–47
  and recurrence, 177
  scars from, 66
  and second cancer, 178, 180
  and sex, 107
  side effects, 5–7, 18–19, 34
Chest X-ray, 32
Children
  choosing guardian for, 220
  deciding to have, 115–17
  emotional adjustment of, 138–40
Chocolate, 48, 57

Cholesterol, 42, 59, 161, 199
Chronic ulcerative colitis, 194
Cisplatin, 77, 78, 87
Citrus fruits, 64
Clitoris
    and arousal, 104, 107
    and hysterectomy, 69
    and pelvic exenteration, 99
    and vulvectomy, 101
Clonidine hydrochloride (Catapres), 158
Clostridium dificile, 82
Coffee, 48, 49
Colon, and fiber, 45–46
Colon cancer, 16, 152, 181
    and alcohol, 48
    coping with surgery and ostomy, 70–72
    and diet, 43, 50, 51, 155
    and exercise, 52
    and fat intake, 38, 45–46
    follow-up care, 32, 33
    genetic legacy and, 127, 128
    and hormone replacement therapy, 153, 155
    prevention and screening for, 94, 193–96
    and second cancer, 178, 183, 188
    warning signs, 198
Colonoscopy, 33, 178, 195
Colostomies
    coping with, 70–72
    and fiber tablets, 47
    and sex, 105–6
Community rating law, 213
Compression garments, 84–85
Compression pump, 84, 85
Condoms, 193
Congestive heart failure, 78
Consolidated Omnibus Budget Reconciliation Act (COBRA), 216–17
Constipation
    and chemotherapy, 77–78
    and fiber, 46
Continent urinary diversion, 69
Cooking tips, 43, 63
Coping magazine, 231
Coping tips, 25–26

Corn, 46
Cortisone medications, 160
Cosmetic surgery, 68
Cough, 31
Co-workers, 203–5
Cream substitutes, 43
Creditor insurance, 219–20
Cruciferous vegetables, 50
Cyclooxygenase, 64
Cytoxan, 118

Dairy products, 43, 51, 160, 192
Decaffeinated coffee, 49
Dehydration, 47, 78, 82
Dentist visits, 30
Depression, 170
    and fatigue, 16
    following treatment, 13–15, 21
    and menopause, 99, 147
    and sex, 107
    treating, 22–23, 172–74
DES ACTion, 234
DES (diethylstilbestrol), 149, 154, 183
Diabetes, 38, 52, 188
Diagnosis
    anniversary of, 8, 12–13
    depression triggered by, 22–23
Diarrhea, 31
    and chemotherapy, 10
    and radiation, 82–83
Diet, 29–30, 38–52, 153
    and alcohol intake, 47–48
    and avoiding future cancer, 180–81
    caffeine in, 48–49
    and calcium, 51–52
    and colostomy, 71
    cutting fat in, 38–45, 55
    and diarrhea, 82–83
    difficulty of maintaining, 55–57
    and dry mouth, 82
    fiber in, 45–47
    and protein, 47
    strategies, 57–59
    and stress, 167–68
    and vitamin supplements, 49–51
Digitalis, 79

Diglycerides, 59
Dignity, 223–24
Digoxin, 79
"Diploid" tumor, 126
Disability insurance, 215, 217, 220
Diuretics, 79
Diverticulitis, 78
Diverticulosis, 46
Divorce, and finances, 222–23
Dizziness, 31
Doctor
    and job discrimination, 209–10
    talking to, about sex, 96–98, 108
    See also Oncologist
Douche, 100
Drivanos, Patricia, 218
Drug abuse, 173
Dry mouth (xerostomia), 81–82
DTIC, 77
Dying
    choice in, 223
    first thoughts about, 3–4
    and survivor support groups, 24

"Ejection fraction" test, 78–79
Electrocardiogram (EKG), 78
Embryo transfer, 119
Emergency fund, 219
Emotions
    and body/mind connection, 164–65
    and coping with scars, 67
    and depression, 172–74
    and family, 134–38
    getting help for negative, 21–25
    informing doctor about, 33
    and loneliness, 169–72
    and stress, 165–69
    and surgery on sex organs, 98–103
    talking about, 15, 25
    when treatments end, 10–15
Employer, 205–8
ENCORE, 233
Endometrial cancer, 21
    and fat intake, 38, 155
    and heredity, 128
    and hormone replacement therapy, 149, 151, 156
    prevention and screening for, 187–88
    and second cancer, 178, 183
    and tamoxifen, 161
Endometriosis, 154
Endorphins, 20, 57–58
Energy level, 16–17
Environment, 37
Epidermal growth factor, 126
Equal Employment Opportunities Commission (EEOC), 210, 212, 237
ERISA, 206
Esophagus cancer, 48, 60, 181
Estate planning, 222
Estrogen
    and breast cancer, 149–50, 155
    in fat cells, 39
    and fiber, 45
    and HDL, 146
    and menopause, 146–47
    and tumor receptor status, 126
Estrogen replacement therapy, 103
    alternatives to, 157–62
    benefits vs. risks of, 145–50, 188
    when not to take, 152–54
    when to take, 155–57
Exercise, 153, 178
    difficulty maintaining, 56–57, 60
    and fatigue, 86
    and future cancer, 181
    for health, 37
    and heart and lung problems, 79
    and hot flashes, 159
    need for, 52–53
    and osteoporosis, 159
    and stress, 166–67
    starting program, 30, 53–55
Explanation of benefits (EOB), 215–16

Facials, 30
Fallopian tubes, 98, 118
Familial adenomatous polyposis syndrome, 195
Family, 14–15
    cancer's effect on, 132–43

Family (*cont.*)
  dependence on, 13
  and job discrimination, 206
  and life insurance, 225
  support groups, 24
Family and Medical Leave Act, 206–7
Fat, 29, 189, 194
  and breast cancer, 40–41, 183
  calories in, 41–42
  as cancer promoter, 38–40, 149, 153
  cutting, 41–45
  digestion, and fiber, 45–46
  "tooth," 58
Fatigue, 172
  and radiation, 85–86
  and sex, 94, 107
  after treatment ends, 16–17
Fecal occult blood test, 199
Federal Rehabilitation Act (1973), 206
Fenretinide (retinoic acid), 186–87
Fertility, 117–23
Fertility drugs, 121, 189
Fever, 31
F. E. Young & Co., 235
Fiber, 78
  and colostomy, 71
  need for, 45–47
  to prevent cancer, 180–81, 194
  supplements, 46, 47
Financial planning, 218–23
Fingernails, 18
Flatulence, 71
Flu, 31
Folate metablism, 48
Folic acid, 64
Follow-up care, 21, 27–36
  developing plan for, 34–35
  difficulty going, 27–28
  preparing for, 28–31
  and recurrence, 177–78
  staying in contact after, 35–36
  what to expect during, 32–33
Food additives, 62–63
Food and Drug Administration, 41, 74
Food cravings, 58

Food diary, 42
Friends
  and follow-up visit, 32
  lost, xiv, 170–72
Fructose, 59
Fruit juices, 82
Fruits, 42, 43, 45, 46, 50, 181
  cooking, 63

Galactose, 192
Gallbladder disesase, 153, 154
Gallstones, 78
Gamete intrafallopian transfer (GIFT), 121
Gas, 31, 34
Gatorade, 82
Genetics, 126–29
  screening, 181–82, 195
Genogram, 129–30
Gestational trophoblastic disease, 80
Gilda Radner Ovarian Cancer Registry, 235
Good Vibrations, 235
Greenwald, Dr. Peter, 40
Guardian, 220
Guilt, 22–23
  and sex, 92
Gynecological reconstruction, 68–69
Gynecologist, 32, 97–98, 108

Hair loss, 5–6, 9
  and sex, 94
Headache, 31
Head cancer, 178
Health and Human Services, Department of, 205
Health care proxy, 222, 223
Health insurance, 212–25
Health maintenance, xiv, 37–65
Health maintenance organization (HMO), 218
Hearing problems, 78
Heartburn, 31
Heart damage
  from chemotherapy, 78–79, 116
  from radiation, 180

Heart disease, 29, 38, 50, 78
  and exercise, 52
  and menopause, 144, 145, 148, 149
Hemoglobin test, 199
HER-2/neu positive, 126
Hereditary Cancer Institute, 236
High-density lipoprotein (HDL), 48, 146, 148
Hodgkin's lymphoma, 109, 155, 156, 178–79, 180
Holland, Dr. Jimmie, 22
Homosexuality, 108
Hormone replacement therapy, 51, 69, 98
  alternatives to, 157–62
  defined, 146–49
  and IVF, 121
  and menopause, 144–45
  risks of, 144–50, 181, 183
  weighing risks, 151–52
  when not to take, 152–54
  when to take, 154–57
Hormones, and diet, 39
Hot flashes, 48, 68, 144, 145, 147, 181
  alternative therapies for, 158–59
  and tamoxifen, 161
Household chores, 142–43
Humor, 25–26, 168
Humor Project, 236
Hypertension, 78, 188
Hyperthyroidism, 81
Hypnosis, 23
Hypothyroidism, 81
Hysterectomy, 15, 39, 40
  and hormone replacement therapy, 145
  and reconstructive surgery, 68–70
  and sex after, 98–99

Ibuprofen, 35, 81
Ice cream, 57–58
Ileostomies, 47
Immune system, 5, 87–88
  and attitude, 19–20
  and beauty treatments, 30
  and dentist visits, 30
  and exercise, 52
  and fat intake, 39
  and follow-up care, 36
  and smoking, 60–61
  and stress, 164–65
  and sun, 62
Imodium, 82
Incontinence, 83
Indigestion, 31
Indoor exercise machines, 55
Infections, 36, 82, 85
Infertility treatments, 119–23
Inflammatory bowel disease, 194
"In-force ledger," 219
Insomnia, 144, 172
Insurance, 212–18
  cancelled, 217
  do's and don'ts, 224–25
  finding help for, 222
Insurance benefits manager, 214–15
Insurance companies
  and infertility treatments, 120
  and job rights, 204–5
  reconstructive surgery, 74
  and restorative surgery and prostheses, 68
  switches, 215, 224
International Association of Laryngectomees, 234
In vitro fertilization (IVF), 119, 120–21, 123
Iron supplements, 29, 194
Isolation, 8, 13, 15, 163, 169–72

Jillian, Ann, xiii
Job Accommodation Network, 208
Job or career
  accommodations, 207–8
  and chemotherapy, 5–6, 7
  discrimination, xiv, 201–12
  and insurance, 8
  loss, and insurance, 216–17
  search, 211–12
  -sharing, 210
  and stress, 167
Journal of the American Medical Association, 155
Journal of the National Cancer Institute, 48

Kidney function, 32
   and chemotherapy, 78, 116
   and radiation, 82
Kinesiology, 64

Labor, Department of, 205
Lady Grace Stores, 233
Large intestine, 45
Larynx cancer, 17, 181
Lawyer, 222
Laxatives, 29
Learning, 171
Lesbians, 108, 235
Let's Face It, 234
Letters, 172
Leukemia, 60, 178
   and pregnancy, 118
Leukemia Society of America, 234
Lhermitte's sign, 18
Life insurance, 8, 202, 219, 225
Lifestyle, 33, 37–65
Liver
   cancer, 48, 181
   disease, 153, 154, 158, 159
   function, 32
Living will, 222, 223–24
Local recurrence, 176
Lomotil, 82
Loneliness, 13, 164, 169–72
Long-term side effects, 35–36
Low-fat diet, 39–41, 180–81, 195
   maintaining, 55–60
   tips for, 43–45
Low-fat substitutes, 44
Lubrin, 104
Lumpectomy, 3–4
   coping with, 76
   side effects from, 80–81
Lumps, 31
Lung
   capacity, 54
   and chemotherapy, 78, 79, 116
Lung cancer, 60, 178, 180
   and diet, 50
   warning signs, 198
Lupus, 74

Lymphatic cancers, 118
Lymphedema, 83–85
   and job, 208–9
   and sex, 107
Lymph nodes
   examination of, 32
   positive, 4–5
   and pregnancy, 125–26
   and radiation, 83–85
   and recurrence, 176
   removal, 36
   signs of spead to, 31
Lymphovascular invasion, 4

McDonald's, 59
Magnetic resonance imaging (MRI), 32, 75, 199
Mammogram, 2, 32, 35, 157, 178, 180
   regular, 185–86, 199
   and silicone implants, 75
Manicures, 30
Mastectomy, 67–68, 90
   prophylactic, 187
   and reconstruction, 73–76
   and sex, 94–95
Masturbation, 108, 111
Mautner Project, 232
Mayonnaise substitutes, 43
Mebestrol acetate (Megace), 158
Medical costs, deducting, 224–25
Medical Information Bureau (MIB), 224
Medical leave, 206–7
Medicare, 217
Medications, 29, 35
Melanoma, 61–62
   and emotions, 165
   and hormone replacement therapy, 154
   prevention and screening for, 196–97
Memory loss, 80
Menopause, 31, 144–62, 183
   and alcohol, 48
   alternative therapies for, 157–62
   and exercise, 52
   and hormone therapy, 146–57
   and hysterectomy, 68

premature, and cancer treatments, 8, 146–47
premature, and pregnancy, 118
and sex, 92, 99
Mental illness, 22
Metabolism, 52
Metastasis, 5, 176
3-methylcholathrene, 46
Microwaving, 63
Migraine headaches, 154
Milex Products, Inc., 235
Moles, 62
Moniliasis, 105
Monounsaturated fats, 41
MOPP (Mustargen, Oncovin, Procarbazine, Prednisone), 118
Mouth, cancer of, 48
Mullan, Dr. Fitzhugh, 15
Music, 169
My Image After Breast Cancer, 233
Myocutaneous flap, 74

Narcotics, 77–78
National Academy of Elder Law Attorneys, 222
National Alliance of Breast Cancer Organizations, 230
National Association of Claims Assistance Professionals, 216
National Association of Insurance Commissioners, 214
National Breast Cancer Prevention Trial, 162
National Cancer Institute, 43, 45, 49–50, 124, 150, 162, 179
National Cancer Institute, Division of Cancer Prevention and Control, 40
National Cancer Survivors Day Foundation, 231
National Coalition for Cancer Survivorship, 15, 210, 216, 229
National Consumer Helpline, 238
National Hospice Organization, 239
National Infertility Network Exchange, 235
National Institutes of Health, 41, 148

National Insurance Consumer Organization, 238
National Lymphedema Network, 232
National Rehabilitation Information Center, 238
National Self-Help Clearinghouse, 238
National Women's Health Network, 155, 232
Natural disastor survivors, 14
Natural killer cells, 52
Nature, 167
Nausea, 28, 31
and chemotherapy, 6, 10
Neck cancer, 60, 81, 178
Neck stiffness, 31
Nelson, Linda, 14
Neuropathy (nerve damage), 77, 116, 139
New England Journal of Medicine, 148
Nicotine patches, 61
Nonprescription drugs, 29
Nonstick pans, 43
Numbness, 11, 77

Obesity
and alcohol, 48
and cancer risk, 38, 153, 155–56
and exercise, 52
Obstetrician, 117
Older women, and sex, 110–12
Oncogene research tests, 126
Oncologist
asking, for support, 31–32
communicating with, 28–31
and estate planning, 222
informing, 33–34
list of questions for, 28–29
and pregnancy, 117
and sex, 96–98, 108, 111–12
staying in touch with, 35–36
Oophorectomy, prophylactic, 190–91
Oral contraceptives, 1, 188, 191
Oral sex, 107, 111
Orgasm, 108
and hysterectomy, 69, 98–99
Orthopedic problems, 54
Osteoarthritis, 52

Osteoporosis, 29, 38, 51, 52, 55
    alternatives to hormone therapy for, 159–60
    and calcium supplements, 152
    and hormone therapy, 156
    and menopause, 144, 145, 148, 149
    screening, 160
    and tamoxifen, 160–62
Ostomy surgery, 16
    living with, 70–72
    and sex, 99
Ovarian cancer, 12, 15, 18, 21, 22, 23, 50, 136, 140, 152, 183
    and chemotherapy, 77, 79
    and diet, 57
    and fat intake, 39
    and fertility drugs, 121
    and follow-up care, 32, 34, 35
    and heredity, 127, 128–29, 190–91
    and hormone replacement therapy, 153, 155
    and job accommodation, 207
    and overweight patient, 40
    pregnancy after, 113, 117, 118
    prevention and screening for, 182, 188–92
    and recurrence, 177
    and second cancer, 178, 188, 194
    sex after, 90, 92, 93–94, 98–99
    side effects of treatment, 87
    warning signs, 198
Ovaries, and hysterectomy, 69
Ovum donation, 122

Pain, 18, 31
    medications, 35
    and radiation treatments, 80–81
    and sex, 103–5, 107
Pancreatic cancer, 49, 60
    and exercise, 52
Papain, 81
Pap smear, 32, 61, 193, 198
Paragoric, 82
Pathology report, 4
Pedicures, 30
Peer support, 24

Pelvic exam, 177
    annual screening, 188, 190, 193
    and follow-up visit, 32
    and overweight patient, 39–40
Pelvic exenteration, 99–100
Pelvic radiation, 82–83
Pepto-Bismol, 82
Perception, 80
Peripheral neuropathy, 18, 54
Personal landmarks, 8–9
Pesticides, 62
Phlebitis, 153
Photon bone density machines, 160
Physical rehabilitation center, 30
Physical therapist, 30, 35
Pickled foods, 63
Pilocarpine, 82
Planning ahead
    and job, 203–4
    and stress, 168
Plastic surgery, 68, 75
"Ploidy" of tumor, 126
Polyps, 193, 194, 195
Polyunsaturated fats, 41
"Portable" insurance, 213
Positive attitude, 25
Poultry, 43
Power of attorney, 222, 223–24
"Preexisting medical condition," 212, 213, 214, 218
Pregnancy and birth, 113–31
    and breast cancer, 124–26
    and decision to have children, 115–17
    and fertility problems, 117–23
Preservatives, 62
President's Committee on the Employment of People with Disabilities, 238
Priorities, 169
Progesterone
    and hormone replacement therapy, 148, 149, 150
    and menopause, 146–47
    receptor status of tumor, 126
Progestin, 145, 156
Prostate cancer, 194

Prostheses, 35, 68
    coping with need for, 67, 73–74
    and sex, 95
Protein, 47
Psychiatrist, 23
Psychologist, 23
Psychotherapy, 16, 141
Pulmonary embolism, 153
Pulmonary fibrosis, 79

Radiation therapy, 3, 4, 16
    and diet, 46
    emotions at end of, 11
    and exercise, 53
    fears during, 7
    pregnancy after, 116, 118–19, 127
    and second cancer, 178, 179, 183
    sex after, 101–2
    side effects from, 66, 76, 79–85
Radner, Gilda, xiii
Rape, 92
Raw-juice therapy, 64
Reconstructive surgery
    breast, 74–76
    gynecological, 68–70
Recovery markers, 18
Rectal examination, 32, 188, 194
Recurrence
    diet and lifestyle to avoid, 37–65
    fears of, 23–24
    and follow-up tests, 32–33
    prevention, xiv
    reasons for, 176–78
    symptoms of, 30–31
    warning signs and screening, 182–99
Red blood cells, 85–86
Regional recurrence, 176
Rehabilitation Services Administration, 238
Reiner, Carl, 168
Relaxation techniques, 23
Remission, 8, 11
Replens, 104
Reproductive endocrinology, 117
Reproductive technology, future, 123
Rest, 16, 86

Restaurants, 42, 63
Résumé, 211
Retinoids, 65
Rheumatoid arthritis, 74
Risk factors
    for breast cancer, 183
    for cervical cancer, 192–93
    for colorectal cancer, 194
    for ovarian cancer, 189
    for skin cancer, 196
    for uterine cancer, 188
Rolin, Betty, xiii
Room freshener, 72
Runowicz, Dr. Sheldon, 1, 3, 4, 6, 8

Sadness, 13, 21, 67, 172, 163–74
Saline implants, 75
Saliva, 81–82
Salpingo-oophorectomy, 40, 99
Saturated fats, 41
Scars, 31
    coping with, 66–88
    and radiation, 80–81
    and sex, 94–95
Scleroderma, 74
Second cancers, 178–80
Self-examination
    for breast cancer, 184
    for skin cancer, 62
Senokot (senna concentrate), 78
Sex, 29, 89–112
    and body image, 93–95
    and breast cancer, 107
    and colostomy, 71–72, 105–6
    drive, diminished, 107–8
    easing into, 106–7
    and hysterectomy, 69, 98–99
    and menopause, 147
    and myth of catching cancer, 91–93
    and older women, 110–12
    and pain, 103–5
    and pelvic exenteration, 99–100
    redefining, 107–8
    and singles, 109–10
    talking to doctor about, 96–98, 108, 111–12

Sex (*cont.*)
  and vaginal stenosis, 101–3
  and vulvectomy, 100–101
  when to begin, 30
Sexual abuse, 92–93
SHARE, 233
Shark cartilage, 64
Shiitake mushroom tea, 64
Sigmoidoscopy, 33, 194–95, 199
Silicone implants, 74–75
"Sing-talk method," 55
Skiing, 54
Skin cancer, 61–62, 178
  prevention and screening for, 196–97
  warning signs, 198
Skin Cancer Foundation, 197, 237
Sleep, 23, 25, 172
Small intestine, 45
Smoking, 37, 38, 48, 193, 194
  and cancer, 60–61
  coach to help quit, 61
  and second cancer, 180
Smoking cessation group, 61
Social Security
  disability, 216
  and divorce, 222–23
Social worker, 23
Society for Assisted Reproductive Technology, 235
Society of Gynecologic Oncologists, 231
Sommers, Tish, 216
Sonogram, 32, 34, 39–40
Sores, 62, 197
Sour cream substitutes, 43
Soybeans, 51, 160
Speech pathologist, 17
Spine, 31
Squamous cell carcinoma, 62, 196
Staph infection, 36
State insurance laws, 213–14, 218
Stent, 100
Stoma, 70, 71
  cleaning and caring for, 72
  sex with, 105–6
Stomachaches, 29

Stools, 46, 82
  sample, 29, 33, 194
Strang Cancer Prevention Center, 237
Stress, 23
  and immunity, 164–65
  limiting, 165–69
Sugar, 57–58
Suicidal thoughts, 173
Sun exposure, 38, 61–62, 180, 196, 197
Sunscreens, 62, 180, 197
Support
  asking doctor for, 31–32
  reaching out for, 20–25
Support groups, 14, 23
  benefits of, 24–25
  and chance members will die, 24
  colostomy, 71
  and depression, 164
  importance of, 165
  resource list, 229–39
  and stress, 169
Surgery
  coping with scars from, 66
  facing effects from, 67–76
Surrogate wombs, 119, 123
Susan G. Komen Breast Cancer Foundation, 237
Sween cream, 83
Swelling, and lymphedema, 84–85
Swimming, 54–55, 70, 159
Symptoms
  listing, for doctor, 29, 30–31
  problems to watch, 31

Talcum powder, 191
Tamoxifen, 103, 158
  and breast cancer, 186
  and menopause, 160–62
Tape recorder, 32
Tax deductions, 224–25
Taxol, 77
Throat cancer, 17, 48, 181
Thromboembolic disease, 161
Thyroid cancer, 178, 180
Thyroid gland scarring, 81

Thyroid medication, 160
Tinnitis, 78
Transdermal estrogen, 154
Trans-fatty acids, 59
Transvaginal color-flow Doppler, 190
Trauma of disease, 14, 21
Treatment, 10–26
   coping tips following, 25–26
   emotions following, 10–15
   See also Chemotherapy; Radiation; and specific illnesses
Trusts, 220, 222
Tubal ligation, 191–92
Tumor marker blood tests, 32
2,000-Year-Old Man, The (Brooks and Reiner), 168

Ultrasound, 75
Unemployment insurance, 217
United Ostomy Association, 72, 232
Urinalysis, 199
Urine specimens, 29
Uterine cancer, 30, 55
   and exercise, 52–53
   and fat intake, 39
   follow-up care, 32
   genetic legacy and, 127
   and hormone replacement therapy, 151–52, 155
   and hormones, 149
   and pregnancy, 117
   prevention and screening for, 187–88
   and second cancer, 178, 179, 194
   sex after, 90, 92–94, 96–99
   warning signs, 198
Uterine fibroids, 154
Uterus, loss of, 68–70

Vagina, removal, 69
   sex after, 98–99
Vaginal atrophy, 103
Vaginal bleeding, 100, 157, 161, 192
Vaginal dilators, 101–3, 157–58
Vaginal dryness, 68, 98
   alternative therapies for, 157–58
   and menopause, 144, 145, 147
   solving problem of, 104–5
Vaginal infection, 105
Vaginal lubrication, 69, 92, 99
   using, 103–4, 105, 157
Vaginal pain, and sex, 103–5
Vaginal reconstruction, 99–100
Vaginal stenosis, 101–3
Vaginal warts, 193
Vaginismus, 105
Vegetable oil, 59
Vegetables, 43, 45, 46, 50, 64, 160, 181
   and calcium, 51
   cooking, 63
Vegetarian diet, 50
Vinblastine, 77
Vincristine, 77
Viruses, 52
Vision, blurred, 31
Visual imagery, 168
Vitamin A, 49, 50, 65
Vitamin C, 49
Vitamin D, 51
Vitamin E, 49
Vitamin supplements, 29, 30, 49–51
Vocational training, 217
Volunteering, 171–72
Vulvar cancer
   follow-up care, 32
   radiation side effects, 83–84
   sex after, 90, 100–101
Vulvectomy
   and reconstructive surgery, 69–70
   sex after, 100–101

Walking, 25, 31, 54, 56, 57, 155, 159
Water aerobics, 54
Water therapy, 167
Weight-bearing exercise, 159
Weight gain, 173
   and breast cancer, 149
   and smoking, 61
Weight gain or loss, sudden, 31
Weight loss, 153, 173, 178
   difficulty of, 55–57

Weight loss (*cont.*)
   and exercise, 52
   for health, 37, 155–56
Wellness Community, 20, 231
Well Spouse Foundation, 236
Where to Write for Vital Records, 129
White blood cell count, 5, 10
Whole grains, 43, 45, 46
Will, 222, 223–24
Wilms's tumor, 180
Winter squash, 50
Women's Health Initiative, 41
World Health Organization, 48

Xandria Foundation, 235
Xerostomia, 81–82
X-rays, 199

Yeast infections, 104
Y-ME, 233
Yoga, 167

Zygote intrafallopian transfer (ZIFT), 121–22